Fiona Marshall is a f...
author with a particu... interest in epilepsy.
She writes regularly for the UK health and
medical press, and has written three books,
Coping Successfully with your Second child,
Coping with Postnatal Depression and *Losing a
Parent*.

The 'Natural Way' series

Increasing numbers of people worldwide are falling victim to illnesses which modern medicine, for all its technical advances, often seems powerless to prevent – and sometimes actually causes. To help with these so-called 'diseases of civilisation' more and more people are turning to 'natural' medicine for an answer. The *Natural Way* series aims to offer clear, practical and reliable guidance to the safest, gentlest and most effective treatments available – and so give sufferers and their families the information they need to make their own choices about the most suitable treatments.

Books in the series:

Allergies
Asthma
Heart Disease

Natural Way

EPILEPSY

FIONA MARSHALL

*Series medical consultants Dr Peter Albright MD
(USA) & Dr David Peters MD (UK)*

Approved by the
AMERICAN HOLISTIC MEDICAL ASSOCIATION
& BRITISH HOLISTIC MEDICAL ASSOCIATION

First Published by Element Books Ltd, 1998
© Vega 2002
Text © Fiona Marshall, 1998

ISBN 1-84333-031-8

A catalogue record for this book is available
from the British Library

Published in 2002 by
Vega
64 Brewery Road
London, N7 9NT

A member of **Chrysalis** Books plc

Visit our website at www.chrysalisbooks.co.uk

Printed in Great Britain
by Butler & Tanner Ltd, Frome and London

Note from the Publisher:
The books in this series are intended for information and guidance only.
They are not intended to replace professional advice, and readers are
strongly urged to consult an experienced practitioner for a proper
diagnosis or assessment before trying any of the treatments outlined.

Contents

List of Illustrations

To all who wrestle with epilepsy

Acknowledgements

First and foremost, grateful thanks to my family for their forbearance while this book was in progress, and in particular to my husband, Peter Cheevers, without whose generosity in looking after our three children the work would not have been done.

I would also like to thank the following for their help: Abi King of the British Epilepsy Association for her general help and the generous use of the EPDATA facility; Caroline Black and Amanda Cummergen of the National Society for Epilepsy, UK; Dr Tim Betts of the Hale Clinic, London; Stefan Ball of the Dr Edward Bach Centre, UK; Dr David Curtain, homeopath; Taj Diora, osteopath; Sino European Clinics; Val Strong of Support Dogs, UK. Special thanks to those who shared their experiences of epilepsy with me, including Cathy Fox, Tina Romano, Emma Shand and Andrew Wise. Thanks also to Michael, who first made me aware of epilepsy.

Introduction

What happens to me during a seizure? What do I look like? How do people think of me? How will it affect me? Will I die? To have epilepsy is to have a whole other identity, which involves managing a huge amount of uncertainty. If your epilepsy is controlled, this other identity may only be revealed to the outside world by your careful and conscious choice. If it is less well controlled, revelation may be involuntary, in the form of a sudden seizure. This lack of control over one's body, this unpredictability, is an aspect of having epilepsy which can be very difficult to live with.

This book aims to outline ways in which it is possible to take more control, and this issue of control has the more relevance because epilepsy is so common. Every day, around 100 people in the UK are told they have epilepsy, while there are about 125,000 newly diagnosed cases each year in the USA. For many people, a diagnosis of epilepsy means drug treatment for life, and has potentially devastating long-term effects on lifestyle, happiness and health.

Conventional medical treatment of epilepsy has traditionally focused on seizure control by drugs – a measure which controls 70–80 per cent of epilepsy. However, while many people are grateful that drug treatment allows them to lead normal lives, side-effects are a problem for many, and, because of this or for other reasons, some may decide not to take their drugs. Some people, too, just don't respond to the best drug treatment.

In cases like these, seizures continue, sometimes interfering with daily life to a disabling extent.

Important as seizure control is, though, in recent years
there has been growing emphasis on overall quality of
life – from people with epilepsy themselves, and from
many medical practitioners, conventional as well as
alternative. There also seems to be a growing feeling that
it is high time that people with epilepsy took more of an
active role and had more of a say in their treatment. In
a nationwide British Epilepsy Association survey
(Perceptions of Epilepsy, and Attitudes Towards Services
and Advice, 1995), 65 per cent of people said that they
wanted to have more choice over their treatment for
epilepsy and 67 per cent wanted a more co-operative
relationship with their doctor. 'Therefore the time seems
ripe for people with epilepsy to take some control over
their position,' says survey leader Professor John Collings, of Leeds Metropolitan University, Leeds, UK. 'Of
course, people need to be armed with accurate information if they are to have an impact on policy makers
and services otherwise they will simply not be heard.'
Professor Collings, who surveyed the attitudes and
experiences of people with epilepsy as part of a BEA
initiative to improve services for people with epilepsy in
the UK, recommends more of a 'holistic approach' which
takes into account people's perceptions of, and attitudes
towards, epilepsy.

It is hoped that this book will go some way towards
helping people to be 'armed with accurate information'.
As well as looking at the conventional treatment options,
the book also explores therapies which are gentle and
natural. Over the past few years there has been a surge
of interest in complementary therapies for epilepsy,
which may help achieve better quality of life for many.
Some people have found that natural remedies appear
to improve their seizure pattern, sometimes dramatically,
sometimes less so. People with epilepsy react in very different ways to complementary therapies, but, generally

speaking, this is an area which, as well as offering therapeutic possibilities, can also be successful in giving people with epilepsy a sense of control over their bodies and their lives. This book aims to provide a starting point to the forms of help available, and where they may be found.

Note: It is particularly important in epilepsy that complementary treatments don't interfere with any existing drug treatment. This isn't really a problem with most therapies, as very few of them will interfere with drug treatments, and indeed, from the holistic point of view, any therapies can work together, complementary and conventional. However, do discuss any alternative treatment with your family doctor or epilepsy specialist first.

What is important is that you should never stop taking your regular medication without medical supervision. Suddenly giving up prescribed drugs can be dangerous in epilepsy, as it can trigger a prolonged seizure (status epilepticus) which may be life-threatening. Also, it is possible that you yourself may feel that now you're taking complementary treatment, you no longer need the conventional kind. Remember that conventional and complementary therapies can, and do, work in harmonious partnership.

This said, it is sometimes possible to reduce epilepsy medication, but this should only be done under the guidance of your doctor. Coming off drugs needs careful thought, as it has other implications than health – for example, if seizures return, you will forfeit your driving licence. Complementary therapies can also provide very useful support during withdrawal if you have been advised by your doctor to decrease medication.

CHAPTER 1

What is epilepsy?

'It's something totally unpredictable which affects my whole life – if I'm out with the pushchair, I have to walk right down the road to the pelican crossing in case I have a seizure trying to cross alone.' – Tina

'It doesn't bother me. I just have to remember to take my medication, that's all, and I have a drug wallet with the days printed out to make it easier.' – Jack

'It's a smell like sulphur which hits me before I have a seizure. That's all I know about my epilepsy.' – Reggie

'It means I lose three days every time I have a seizure – a day and a half building up, with really bad headaches and not being able to speak straight, and then a day or so afterwards of feeling really depressed.' – Anna-Maria

Epilepsy is a complex subject which raises several questions about how the brain works, and its links with emotions, thoughts, the memory and personality. Epilepsy occurs when the brain, normally a well-ordered organ managing thousands of tasks on a daily basis, suddenly halts and throws the whole system into confusion – rather like one car stopping suddenly on a fast-moving roundabout.

Epilepsy happens either because part of the brain has become damaged in some way, or because the person is genetically predisposed to it. Epilepsy, derived from the ancient Greek, means 'to be seized by forces from without'. It's now known that these forces are very much within, and epilepsy is usually defined as a tendency to have recurrent seizures (fits) caused by abnormal electrical activity in the brain, which, if untreated, can interfere with normal living with disastrous effect. In one sense, there is no such thing as epilepsy, as it is a general term applied to many different people with many different conditions – a very wide spectrum of brain conditions can cause epilepsy. This is why some medical textbooks refer to 'the epilepsies'. Epilepsy is usually viewed as a symptom of underlying brain disorder, rather than as a disease in its own right, and 'should perhaps be considered no more than a stereotyped reaction of the brain to a variety of stresses', say British neurologists Anthony Hopkins and Richard Appleton (see page 120 for details of their book, *Epilepsy, The Facts*).

About the brain (1)

To understand epilepsy and seizures, it is necessary to have an idea of how the brain works, and how it is constructed.

Normal brain function is made possible by millions of tiny electrical charges passing between nerve cells in the brain and to all parts of the body. In a seizure, this normal pattern may be interrupted by intermittent bursts of electrical energy that are much more intense than usual. These 'storms' affect the delicate systems in charge of the brain's electrical energy, and may affect a person's consciousness, bodily movements or sensations for a short time. Normal brain function cannot return until the electrical bursts subside.

Basically, the brain is divided into two halves (hemispheres) which are linked in the middle. The right half controls the left-hand side of the body and is responsible for the sense of music, art and recognition of faces. The left half controls the right-hand side and is responsible for understanding and processing language, the sense of time, logical thought and mathematical thought. It's a fantastically delicate and precise instrument which controls a complex interweaving of emotions, senses and bodily feelings, all of which can be disrupted by seizure activity.

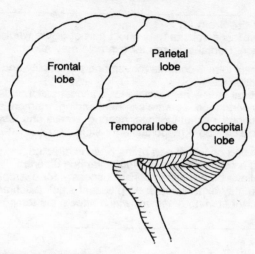

Fig. 1 The four lobes of the brain

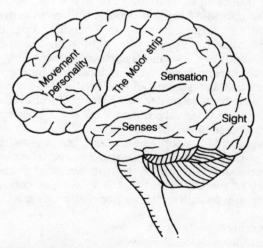

Fig. 2 What the brain controls

About the brain (2)
  An epileptic seizure may affect part of or the whole of
the brain. Partial seizures for example may affect:

- Frontal lobe – controls movement, personality and
  emotions.
- Parietal lobe – responsible for body sensations.
- Temporal lobe – controls understanding, memories,
  emotions, sexual feelings, hearing, smells and tastes.
- Occipital lobe – responsible for sight.

Depending on which part of the brain is affected, the person
having a seizure may experience various different
sensations before losing consciousness – for example, a
person may experience an unpleasant smell (such as
sulphur) if starting a seizure which affects the temporal
lobe.

Who has epilepsy?

Epilepsy is the most common serious brain disorder until
old age, affecting an estimated one in 200 people globally
– that's some 40–55 million people. Epilepsy occurs more
frequently in certain cultures. In Tanzania, 4 per cent of
the population has epilepsy, thought to be due to genetic
factors. Epilepsy is slightly more common in men,
especially certain types such as temporal lobe epilepsy.
Research has also suggested that this is because men are
more prone to head injury. But these cultural and gender
variations are relatively minor – on the whole epilepsy
is no respecter of sex or race.

   Epilepsy affects people of any age, but is usually diagnosed in childhood. There is also a surge in epilepsy in
the over-sixties – a survey by the National Society for
Epilepsy in the UK found that it is twice as common in
older people as in the British population as a whole.

Is it curable?

Cure implies a disease. However, epilepsy is not viewed
as a disease, but a long-term disorder with an underlying

cause, which may be controlled, not cured, by drugs. In a few people, this underlying cause is another illness which may be cured. In a few others, surgery may be able to remove the cause of the epilepsy (see page 53).

This may sound unduly discouraging, and many patients (and doctors) do feel that they are stuck with epilepsy for life. However, the good news is that some people do appear to go into remission (i.e. a period free from seizures) – in other words, their epilepsy appears to get better of its own accord. According to one long-term study from Olmstead County, USA, twenty years after diagnosis about 50 per cent of people had been seizure-free without anti-epileptic drugs for at least five years.

This kind of research obviously shouldn't be seen as an inducement to throw all your drugs away. But it can be viewed as encouraging if you wish to try complementary therapies. It is sometimes possible to regard a regular drug regime as a kind of 'safety blanket' and to allow it to limit exploration of therapies which could enhance your lifestyle and well-being (even if they don't cure your epilepsy). Knowing that epilepsy sometimes seems to get better is a good reason for trying complementary therapies which might, in some cases, help you towards an improvement in health.

How symptoms vary

One of the hallmarks of epilepsy is the many different forms it can take. It also varies widely in severity. Epilepsy can occur as a condition on its own, or may accompany other conditions affecting the brain, such as cerebral palsy, mental retardation and autism.

Sometimes, before a diagnosis of epilepsy has been made, people may wonder what is happening to them as they experience a range of symptoms which can be confusing or frightening. Symptoms people have complained of include headaches, feeling exhausted, dizziness or extreme vertigo, nausea, feelings of losing control, fighting to keep conscious, lost time or 'blackouts', feeling 'spaced out' or 'odd', or experiencing odd smells such as gas, sulphur or something rotting. These have been experienced singly (i.e. just headaches) or grouped together (i.e. smelling an odd smell *and* feeling giddy and sick).

The main symptoms of epilepsy itself – and what your doctor relies on in order to diagnose epilepsy – are different kinds of recurrent seizures (fits). Diagnosis of epilepsy can be difficult, and must be made by a competent doctor (see page 46). However, seizures can be described as attacks in which consciousness and/or motor activity is interrupted. These may take several forms – the best known is the convulsive seizure, in which consciousness is lost and the person may fall to the ground, body jerking. However, there are many other kinds – for example, the person may suddenly fall to the ground but not lose consciousness, or there may be no more than twitching or jerking of one limb or of the body. Seizures can be even less noticeable than this, and the interrupted consciousness may show as no more than staring and inattention, which are easily mistaken for daydreaming. For a full discussion of seizure types, see pages 12–22.

What epilepsy is not
Historically, there are question marks about where neurology ends and psychiatry begins in epilepsy, but at this point it is probably worth stating what epilepsy is not:

- Epilepsy is not a mental illness such as depression, although psychological factors may play a part in people's experience of epilepsy.
- It is not a psychiatric disorder.
- Neither is it an infectious disease which can be 'caught' like, say, measles.

Epilepsy and behaviour problems
As with anyone, behavioural problems can occur for reasons quite unconnected with epilepsy! However, some people who care for those with epilepsy, especially parents, have found this area extremely distressing. According to a survey in the UK by the British Epilepsy Association called *Caring together in epilepsy*, carers have found the link between behaviour problems and epilepsy highly important, often overlooked and an area where it is often hard to get information and help. The survey suggested three main types of behaviour:

- Behaviour caused by seizures – sometimes seizures can appear to be similar to difficult behaviours. Normal brain functions are suspended, and the person may have no awareness of what he or she is doing.
- Behaviour caused by medication, especially if the dose is too high or too low. For example, it is possible for a person to become 'intoxicated' on too high a dose, and to act out of character.
- Behaviour independent of seizures or medication. In this case, more questions need to be asked about why it is happening, and whether the person may be communicating a need, or otherwise expressing something which he or she cannot verbalize.

The BEA recommends seeking help from your family doctor, epilepsy specialist or specialist epilepsy nurse, and from local psychological and psychiatric services.

Cognitive (higher thinking) problems
Many people with epilepsy are of normal and above average intelligence. In some cases, underlying brain dysfunction can affect areas of intelligence, such as language, leading to added difficulties such as communication problems, which may be especially noticeable around the time of a seizure. And, because they can't easily verbalize their feelings, a few people with language difficulties may have difficulty controlling

their anger in an emotional situation. If these problems aren't identified, a person may unjustly be labelled as simply slow or troublesome.

There is a link between epilepsy and learning disability. About 30 per cent of people with a learning disability have epilepsy; and, in those with a severe learning disability, the number of people with epilepsy increases to 80 per cent. Underlying brain damage or dysfunction can cause both. Again, medication can also make people drowsy, and so less mentally alert.

History of epilepsy

Epilepsy, once known as the sacred disease, has been regarded as a mark both of divine inspiration and of possession by the devil, and attributed to several famous figures including Socrates, Julius Caesar, Alexander the Great, the apostle Paul, Joan of Arc, Napoleon, Dostoevsky, Flaubert, Byron, Edward Lear and van Gogh (though later medical research suggests he may in fact have suffered from porphyria).

Epilepsy itself goes back as far as man himself. Prehistoric man probably had experience of epilepsy and may even have tried to cure it by trephining (or trepanning), or making a hole in the skull. There is also evidence that it was known to the Mesopotamian civilization, when it was thought to be caused by Sin, the god of the moon.

Hippocrates (460–377 BC) was the first to insist that epilepsy originated from the brain, and attacked the charlatans who favoured magical explanations. The ancient Greek physicians favoured a relatively staid regimen of diet, drugs and certain set routines. For example, a typical day for a patient might have comprised regular hours and meals, vinegar and honey drinks and other dietary measures, regular exercise such as taking long walks along straight routes, ending in a bath followed by a head, neck and hand massage.

Set against this mild regime were a whole host of more aggressive and colourful treatments which persisted for several centuries – anything from shaving the person's head, to rubbing him with the genitals of a seal or cauterizing him.

Beliefs continued to range from the crude to the bizarre well into the nineteenth century. Even as late as 1880, castration was a medically recommended treatment to cure the masturbation believed to be the root cause of epilepsy.

For anyone interested, Owsei Temkin's classic book *The Falling Sickness* (see page 120) provides a very full history of epilepsy throughout the ages.

Cost of epilepsy

The annual cost of epilepsy in the UK was estimated by a recent study by the National Society of Epilepsy and the Institute of Neurology, London, as £1,930 million (pounds sterling). The cost of direct care is only around 60 per cent of the total. Around 70 per cent of the care is related to unemployment and mortality caused by active epilepsy.

Mortality and SUDEP

It may come as an unpleasant shock to realize that epilepsy is still a very serious, even life-threatening condition. The risk of premature death in people with epilepsy is two to four times greater than that of the general population, especially among children, young adults and in the first ten years of diagnosis. One study from the University of Minnesota studied a group of more than 4,000 and put the average age of death as forty-two in men and forty in women.

Figures vary, but accidents probably account for about 5 per cent of these early deaths, especially drowning, head injury and traffic accidents. Suicide (which tends to be more common in people with epilepsy) is thought to account for a further 5–10 per cent. Other common causes of death include brain tumour, status epilepticus (prolonged seizures), epilepsy-related conditions, respiratory problems and heart problems. Status epilepticus alone is the cause of between 22,000 and 42,000 deaths in the US each year, according to research from the Mayo Clinic in Rochester, Minnesota.

One rather mysterious cause of death relates to sudden unexplained death in epilepsy (SUDEP), which is most common between the ages of twenty and fifty, and which has been blamed for 5–15 per cent of deaths. In the UK, the number of SUDEP deaths a year is thought to be between 200 and 500, though few doctors are actually aware of SUDEP. Another American study suggested an annual mortality rate of one SUDEP for every 370 people with epilepsy in the community.

Why SUDEP should be a particular problem among people with epilepsy is not clear. Many explanations have been suggested, including the long-term effects of anti-epileptic drugs, the effect of seizures on the heart

---

SUDEP – Am I at risk?
This is an extremely distressing prospect, and one which research is not yet able to clarify. However, certain risk factors seem linked with SUDEP:

- Being a young man and having tonic-clonic seizures which are not controlled by medication
- Not taking medication correctly or regularly
- Being alone during seizures
- Alcoholism

Lacking specific medical recommendations, the following general guidelines are recommended:

- Staying with someone during a seizure and for twenty minutes afterwards to ensure that he or she is breathing smoothly (some relatives, carers or friends may, if they feel they have particular cause for concern, want to learn mouth-to-mouth resuscitation)
- Getting seizures under control as far as possible
- Not stopping anti-epileptic drugs suddenly
- Taking medication regularly

and unwitnessed seizures, but more studies are needed to identify the cause clearly.

Depressing as this may be, it gives all the more reason for people with epilepsy to do what they can to maximize their quality of life. 'Leading a normal life is very important,' says Dr Stephen Brown, a well-known epilepsy specialist and former chairman of the British Epilepsy Association. 'Dealing with the risk of SUDEP is just part of the package.'

CHAPTER 2

Types of epilepsy and seizures

While everyone's experience of epilepsy is individual, epilepsy and seizures can be classified into certain different types.

What is the difference between epilepsy and seizures?

Epilepsy is usually described as the tendency of the brain to produce sudden, repeated bursts of electrical energy that disrupt other brain functions. Epilepsy is also usually viewed as a symptom and not a disease as such – a symptom of underlying brain damage or disorder.

Seizures are signs that epilepsy is present, and can broadly be described as attacks which disrupt consciousness or activity.

Having just one seizure by itself does not necessarily mean you have epilepsy – most doctors will wait until you have had at least two seizures before making a diagnosis. Illness or severe head injury can affect the brain enough to produce a single seizure, and everyone has what's known as a 'seizure threshold' – a certain sensitivity to seizures which means that anyone can experience a seizure, given appropriate conditions such as excess use of alcohol. In fact, around one in twenty people have a single seizure at some point in their lives. Research from the UK suggests that six out of ten people will have a second seizure within twelve months, while other research from the USA puts this figure lower, about three to four people out of ten. When seizures continue to occur, for unknown reasons or because of an underlying problem, then the condition is usually referred to as **epilepsy** or (especially in the USA) **seizure disorder.**

Types of epilepsy

Epilepsy is a very general umbrella term for many different conditions. In the broadest sense, epilepsy is usually divided into:

- **Symptomatic epilepsy,** when seizures are thought to be, as the name implies, symptoms of some underlying structural abnormality in the brain.
- **Idiopathic epilepsy,** when seizures are not thought to be symptoms of underlying brain disease. Idiopathic means 'of unknown cause', and seizures in idiopathic epilepsy are thought to be because a person is constitutionally predisposed to them.

Some types of epilepsy are more common than others, and the following three boxes give examples.

Photosensitive epilepsy
Only a minority of people with epilepsy are photosensitive, which means they react with seizures to sensory stimuli such as flickering sunlight, strobe lights, television, videos and computers. (See page 32 for more on this type of epilepsy.)

Temporal lobe epilepsy (TLE)
This is one of the most common forms of epilepsy, and is slightly more prevalent in men. TLE is another way of looking at *complex partial seizures* (see below) which originate in the temporal lobe.

The temporal lobes, situated at either side of the brain, are vital to the sense of identity which many of us take for granted. They contain many of the functions which combine to create our sense of 'who I am' – memory, emotions and information. The temporal lobes are also involved with receiving sound and smell and with the production of speech and other everyday functions which we rely on. These functions are invaded when seizure activity takes place, which is why the start of seizures (the aura) involves the distortion of many everyday feelings about time, memory, perception, vision and our sense of ourselves. Auras vary a great deal but may include a churning feeling in the stomach, feeling sick, flushing, sweating, going pale, chewing, swallowing or lip smacking. Changes in perception are also common – things appear larger or smaller than before – as are hallucinations and memory distortions.

'I'll be doing some quite ordinary activity when I start feeling that this has all happened before, that it's all happening just as it did the last time and that everything is going to take a certain set course that I can't change,' says Ivan, a twenty-nine-year-old artist. 'As this feeling becomes deeper and I know I can't escape, I start feeling terrified. My last conscious sensation is usually starting to hear a far-off bell ringing, and smelling some unidentifiable smell – at the time, the smell is quite clear but I can never remember what it is afterwards, some fusty, burning smell but I can't identify it fully before I fall unconscious.'

All this is why TLE brings into sharper focus the meaning of having epilepsy – the loss of identity that occurs, of everyday functions being suspended without the person's consent. 'It's as if somebody suddenly undressed you in public,' explains Betty, a forty-five-year-old gardener. 'You're suddenly stripped of your identity on both a social and a personal level. It's not too extreme to say it's a kind of rape, a rape of your consciousness.'

Syndromes of epilepsy

There are many different syndromes of epilepsy, involving different types of seizures, and often beginning in childhood, such as **West syndrome**, which usually involves long-term problems with learning disability and continuing seizures. **Lennox-Gastaut syndrome** starts a little later and is often associated with learning difficulties. **Rasmussen's syndrome** is when part of the brain becomes inflamed and the inflammation slowly spreads (focal encephalitis), also resulting in epilepsy.

Nocturnal (sleep) epilepsy

Some people only experience seizures in their sleep (daytime as well as night-time sleep). They may only know they have had a seizure if they wake up in the morning feeling extra tired, or with signs such as muscle stiffness or with the insides of their cheeks bitten.

Sometimes sleep seizures can be treated with an increased dose of medication in the evening, which you should discuss with your doctor before trying. Regular sleep habits can also help reduce the occurrence of nocturnal seizures.

Seizures

What happens in a seizure?

In an epileptic seizure (fit), normal brain activity is interrupted by brain cells 'firing' much faster than usual. This firing is also 'explosive', producing a bizarre and rather chaotic appearance on the EEG. This may result in various altered states of consciousness, and sometimes consciousness is lost altogether.

Because the brain is so complex, and controls so many different functions, seizures can disrupt many normal aspects of a person, such as personality, mood, memory, sensations and movement. This explains why seizures take so many different forms – for example, the person may stand quite motionless, or just continue with what he or she was doing, or wander off, without showing any dramatic signs of what is going on in the brain inside. Or the seizure may come and go so quickly that no one, not even the person affected, is aware of it.

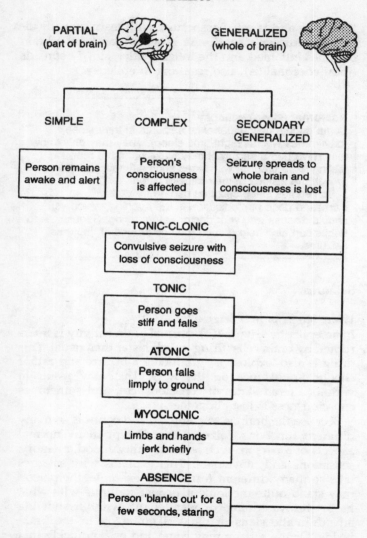

Fig. 3 Seizure types

Types of seizure

Types of epileptic seizure have been redefined by the International League Against Epilepsy, resulting in the International Classification of Seizures, which is most commonly used when describing seizures.

There are around forty different types of seizure, but basically seizures today are divided into two main kinds: **generalized**, where the whole brain is affected and consciousness is lost, and **partial** (or **focal**), where only part of the brain is affected. Seizures as defined by the International League Against Epilepsy are usually classified as follows:

Generalized

- **Tonic-clonic:** The generalized convulsive seizure ('grand mal') is the most common form of epileptic seizure and affects 60 per cent of people with epilepsy. In this type of seizure, the person may go rigid and fall down, sometimes with an involuntary high cry which is caused by air being forced out of the lungs and through the larynx in spasms. The muscles then relax and stiffen alternately, causing the person to jerk in convulsions. This can be distressing to watch, as the person may breathe with difficulty (because the respiratory muscles are also involved in the stiffening process), go blue in the face, foam at the mouth, bite the inside of the cheek or tongue, grunt or be incontinent. However, the person affected is unaware of what is happening, though they may feel very weary or confused when they come round, and may also sometimes be hurt if they hit themselves when falling, or injure themselves against some object on the ground.
- **Tonic:** The person's muscles stiffen and again he or she may fall to the ground, though there is no jerking.
- **Atonic** (or drop attacks): The person may fall suddenly to the ground because of a sudden loss of muscle tone.

- **Myoclonic:** These seizures involve sudden muscle jerks – for example, the head may suddenly nod, or there may be abrupt jerking of the arms and/or legs. Myoclonic attacks may happen on their own or with other generalized seizures. If myoclonic attacks take place in young children they are generally called infantile spasms or 'salaam attacks'. The child's whole body is involved as he or she is thrown forward with their arms up.
- **Absence:** Absence seizures ('petit mal') are common in children, and may often be mistaken for daydreaming. What happens is that the person 'tunes out' for a few seconds as their consciousness is briefly interrupted by abnormal brain activity, though the only signs may be blank staring, blinking, chewing movements, head-turning or other subtle signs such as a tiny dribble of saliva. This kind of seizure can pass unnoticed by everyone, including the person affected, who is not aware that he or she has been 'absent' from conversations or events for a few seconds.

Partial/focal seizures

Partial (or focal) seizures are limited to a certain part of the brain, and consciousness may be affected, but not lost.

- **Simple partial seizures:** These seizures affect a small area of the brain and the person stays awake without consciousness being affected. Simple partial seizures often mark the start of some other form of seizure, for example spreading over the whole brain so that a generalized tonic-clonic seizure is the result. Hence, the aura of a generalized tonic-clonic seizure is also a simple partial seizure.
- **Complex partial seizures:** These are seizures in which consciousness is affected, and when a larger area of the brain is involved. The complex partial seizure spreads, quickly or slowly, and may cut the person

off from the outside world altogether.

The person may experience strange sensations depending on which of the brain's four lobes is affected:

- *In temporal lobe seizures*, the person may have strong emotional experiences, such as fear or terror. Another feeling is of intense *déjà vu* (the feeling that this has all happened before), or, conversely, *jamais vu*, when familiar surroundings and objects appear strange. People affected may 'see' scenes from their past unfolding before their eyes, or have other hallucinations, or forget where they are and what they are doing. They may also experience strong smells or tastes, or, if the speech area of the brain is affected, may speak unintelligibly or be unable to speak. All these feelings are very intense, much more so than our everyday state, and sometimes may be so far removed from it that the people affected have great difficulty describing them afterwards.

- *In frontal lobe seizures*, there may be twitching or jerking of the arms or legs, or involuntary eye movements.

- *In parietal lobe seizures*, there may be tingling or pins and needles in some part of the body, for example down one side.

- *In occipital lobe seizures*, the person may see flashing lights for a few seconds.

A complex partial seizure may also involve automatic behaviour (also known as an *automatism*) in which the people affected wander about, sometimes continuing with actions they were engaged in before the seizure started. They may look purposeful but in fact they have no awareness of what they are doing, and, once the seizure is over, no memory of it. Their actions are usually simple and stereotyped (such as lip-smacking or pulling at clothes) but may be more complicated (such as undressing and putting themselves to bed).

Jacksonian epilepsy
John Hughlings Jackson (1835–1911) was a brilliant and
dedicated doctor widely known as the 'father' of British
neurology. His work paved the way for much epilepsy
research to come. Jackson described what are today
known as **simple partial seizures**, and for this reason they
are still sometimes referred to as Jacksonian seizures.

- **Secondary generalized seizures:** This is when the
  seizure spreads over both halves of the brain so that
  the person loses consciousness and passes into a generalized tonic-clonic seizure. Again, this may happen
  very fast, or more slowly. If it is slow, the patient may
  have a warning ('aura').
- **Status epilepticus:** This is when seizures occur in
  rapid succession and the person remains unconscious
  in the brief intervals between seizures. This is potentially an extremely dangerous condition, as the person
  risks severe brain damage or even death from oxygen
  shortage to the brain. Treatment involves injecting
  anti-epileptic drugs either into the muscles or the
  veins.

Seizures – a fact of life
For many, seizures are still a fact of life despite all that drug
treatment can do. According to the results of a nationwide
survey of more than 4,300 adults with epilepsy:

- 41 per cent have less than one seizure a year.
- 36 per cent have 1–12 seizures a year.
- 23 per cent have more than one seizure a month.

('Living with epilepsy: a patient's viewpoint' was conducted
by the independent market research company AGB Taylor
Nelson, 1994, in conjunction with the British Epilepsy
Association, and sponsored by The Wellcome Foundation
Ltd.)

Non-epileptic attacks (NEAs)

These may look like epileptic seizures to the bystander, but are different in that brain activity is not affected – if the affected person were to have an EEG during the attack, it would be normal. These attacks tend to take place for strong psychological reasons, and can be described as extreme forms of panic attacks or 'cut-off' mechanisms, when seizures are produced as a response to intense stress. They are sometimes called 'pseudo-seizures' but the person is usually very genuine in not being able to control what is happening. Obviously the person cannot be treated with anti-epileptic drugs but should seek medical help, often in terms of referral to a psychologist or psychiatrist. Support from epilepsy organizations or through epilepsy self-help groups can also be useful (see pages 116–19).

Febrile convulsions

Non-epileptic convulsions can occur in babies and young children when their bodies are unable to cope with a sudden high temperature. A tendency to febrile convulsions often runs in families, and the child commonly grows out of it by around age four to five.

Fainting

Fainting (syncope in medical language) occurs when the brain falls short of blood, sometimes as a result of standing for long periods. Occasionally, faints can be confused with seizures – for example, jerking of the limbs can occur as a result of blood shortage to the brain, especially if the person is propped up. Also, in some partial seizures, the person may feel symptoms similar to those of faintness.

Hyperventilation

Hyperventilation, or overbreathing, is when a person feels he is not getting enough air and so breathes too deeply or too quickly. The result is feeling giddy and experiencing tingling, and even spasms of the limbs. Breathing into a paper bag for a few minutes usually helps.

Migraine and epilepsy

A strong relationship between epilepsy and migraine has long been suspected, but has never before been systematically demonstrated. Now, research shows that people with epilepsy are more than twice as likely to develop migraine headaches, according to a study of nearly 2,000 patients done at Columbia's School of Public Health and the Albert Einstein College of Medicine, USA.

Migraine resembles some forms of seizure in that it may start with an aura or warning such as visual disturbances or tingling in the face or arm, as in a simple partial seizure (to make things more complicated, it's not uncommon to have a splitting headache after a seizure). An EEG will show that brain waves sometimes behave in similar ways during a migraine aura and an epileptic seizure. But there are established differences between migraine and epilepsy:

- In migraine, consciousness is hardly ever lost.
- The disturbances in vision are different in migraine (typical are seeing bright light around objects or losing all or part of your vision). In epilepsy, visual disturbances may be of flashing lights or all kinds of individual hallucinations.
- Any tingling tends to spread slowly up the arm in migraine, and quickly in seizures.

CHAPTER 3

Causes of epilepsy and triggers of seizures

Many people may never find out why they have epilepsy. In up to 70 per cent of cases there is no obvious cause. And, given our natural urge to seek out explanations for what happens to us, and to understand cause and effect in our lives, it can be hard to accept this 'up in the air' diagnosis. (Indeed, whether the cause is known or not, many find it hard to accept a diagnosis of epilepsy at all.)

As new research proceeds apace, however, scientists are learning ever more about why epilepsy happens. New scanning techniques and genetic research offer new explanations, and the hope of new treatments in the future.

On a more immediate level, people with epilepsy may be much more concerned to find out what triggers seizures on a day-to-day basis in their particular case. There are definitely some situations in which seizures are more likely, though, as with many aspects of epilepsy, this can be highly individual. Whatever the cause, better understanding of personal triggers does give more chance of controlling your epilepsy.

Causes of epilepsy

Causes of epilepsy
Common causes of epilepsy are:

- Inherited brain disease such as tuberous sclerosis (or epiloia, a rare congenital disorder in which the brain and other organs develop overgrowths which can interfere with the central nervous system).
- Inherited epilepsies such as primary generalized epilepsy.
- Birth trauma – for example, lack of oxygen (anoxia) during the birth.
- Head trauma resulting from accidents, such as car accidents, gunshot wounds, sports accidents, falls and blows. The more severe the injury, the greater the risk of developing epilepsy.
- Problems with the unborn baby's developing brain, sometimes thought to be caused by injury or illness to the pregnant woman.
- Infections, such as meningitis, viral encephalitis, lupus erythematosus and, less frequently, mumps, measles, diphtheria and others.
- Poisoning, such as lead poisoning or aluminium toxicity, or chemical injury to the brain.
- Alcohol poisioning in particular is more common than might be suspected – more than 5,000 people each year are reported to suffer seizures caused by excess alcohol.
- So-called recreational drugs such as Ecstasy or cocaine.
- Blood chemical abnormalities such as low calcium, magnesium or glucose.
- Brain tumours such as gliomas (malignancies in the glial tissue which connects nerve cells and fibres) or meningiomas (a tumour which occurs as a separate growth).
- Stroke (the most common cause of epilepsy in older people).

Head trauma and epilepsy
Work by Professor Bryan Jennett of Glasgow in the UK has pinpointed three main factors most likely to result in epilepsy after injury to the head. These are:

- Length of post-traumatic amnesia. This is the period after the accident when, though conscious, people are not really 'taking in' outside events and have no memory of them later. The longer this amnesia lasts (more than twenty-four hours) the more likely epilepsy is to result.
- Signs which might indicate neurological disturbance, such as changes in the reflexes.
- How much tearing or damage is done to the dura, or membrane covering the brain.

Professor Jennett found that if all three factors were present, there was a 40 per cent risk of developing epilepsy, as opposed to about 2 per cent if not.

Genetic links

Epilepsy is inherited in only a minority of cases. Sometimes, this means that only a *tendency* to epilepsy may be inherited – **not** that people with epilepsy automatically pass it on to their children. For example, abnormal EEG patterns show in 40 per cent of brothers and sisters of children who have epilepsy – even though these siblings don't have seizures themselves. (If you are planning a family and are concerned about the prospect of a child inheriting epilepsy, ask to be referred to a genetic counsellor. Genetic counsellors are trained in genetics and psychology and can help assess the *risk* of passing on epilepsy to a child, though they can't tell you in advance whether a baby will definitely inherit the disorder or not. Working with you, a genetic counsellor creates a comprehensive medical family tree with as many details as possible of all diseases and disorders suffered by your blood relations.)

In fact, everyone inherits a certain susceptibility to

seizure (called your 'seizure threshold'), but in varying degrees, and individual sensitivity to seizures is one of the issues under research at the moment. At the Montreal Neurological Institute, Canada, a pioneering organization in epilepsy research, scientists are looking at how much stimulus the neurons can take before responding with a seizure. Experiments have shown that neurons which receive mild electrical stimulation become increasingly more sensitive to the point where they become prone to seizures. In the same way, the neurons' ability to resist seizures can be impaired by head injuries from, say, cycling or car accidents. By studying stimulus in this way, scientists hope to get a clearer picture of where the genes end and the environment begins. How much sensitivity to seizures is inherited, and how much is due to environmental factors, may be a key question in deciding on future treatments and prevention for epilepsy.

Genetic research – epilepsy genes discovered
Scientists have also succeeded in isolating genes implicated in epilepsy, something which may affect treatment in the long-term future:

- A team at the Institute of Biology in Montpellier, France, identified the first gene known to cause an idiopathic epilepsy. It is linked with a rare form of epilepsy called *benign neonatal familial convulsions*, which affects newborns but disappears by three months.
- Researchers at the pharmaceutical company Novartis Pharma AG, Basel, Switzerland, isolated the gene for one of the most important substances in the brain, the GABA-B receptor, which helps stop brain cells firing uncontrollably (as in a seizure). The discovery may have key implications for future treatments for epilepsy.
- Researchers at Stanford University in California and

the University of Helsinki in Finland believe they have found a gene which leads to a rare form of epilepsy, progressive myoclonus epilepsy.

Causes of epilepsy – the future at the Montreal Neurological Institute (MNI)

The Montreal Neurological Institute, Canada, was largely founded by the American-born Wilder Penfield (1891–1976), a specialist in neurosurgery who emigrated to Canada. Today, MNI leads the world in the field of neurosurgery, and is also an internationally famous centre for epilepsy research. Subjects under research include:

- *Neural dysgenesis:* This is something which can occur naturally in the unborn baby – that is, it is not caused by trauma or by sudden lack of oxygen in the brain. It is a neural malformation which may happen as the embryo develops. This means that some epilepsy may occur due to problems with the developing brain which happen while the baby is still in the womb, and, obviously, if scientists can discover more about how this happens, prevention of epilepsy might be possible in some cases.

- *How seizures affect neurotransmitters:* Researchers are examining how seizures affect neurotransmitters, the chemical substances that relay nerve messages from cell to cell throughout the nervous system. This is a specialized, minute form of research which takes place at molecular level. By discovering how seizures affect neurotransmitters, it might be possible to create drugs which work at transmitter level to halt seizure activity.

- *Neurotrophic factors:* Neurotrophins are proteins that help neurons to grow and survive. Too many or too few neurotrophins can be harmful. Researchers believe that they can harness neurotrophins to treat serious neurological diseases. This could be a possibility for treating brain damage associated with epilepsy.

Seizure triggers

Some people, although not all, find that certain factors trigger seizures. Certain triggers are more common – stress and emotional upset, lack of sleep, illness, excess alcohol, drugs – while others are more individual, and may vary widely.

Stress

Stress is **the** outstanding trigger of seizures for many people with epilepsy. Stress can take many forms but can be due to pressures at work, lack of money, emotional upsets or confrontations, or ongoing problems with a relationship. Fear, anger and excitement have been pinpointed as specific seizure triggers. One man's seizures returned for a while when he was afraid his girlfriend would find out about a promising new flirtation in his life; the situation was compounded by his anger at himself for not being able to handle this state of affairs. Another man found underground trains claustrophobic and had three seizures on different occasions when travelling to work, after which he took the bus. Another man had a seizure while watching an exciting football match, and, incidentally, after having one beer too many with his friends (see **Excess alcohol**, below).

Of course this doesn't mean that people with epilepsy must strive to live a bland life from which the unexpected and challenging is rigorously excluded – boredom too can be a seizure trigger! But, often in combination with other factors, stress can bring on seizures, and some people may need to take extra steps in order to learn how to handle stressful situations in their lives. There's more on this on pages 81–94.

Lack of sleep

As with stress, no one would wish this to become a tyranny, with the threat of a seizure held over your head if you go to bed half an hour later than usual. However, lack of sleep is a known trigger factor in seizures, as it has been shown to change the brain's patterns of electrical activity. In fact, for some EEG tests, patients are asked to attend having had only a few hours' sleep the night before, to make the recording of abnormal brainwave patterns more likely. As with other triggers, each person has to find the right balance of sleep for him or herself.

Illness

A high temperature may make people more prone to seizures, though this isn't to be confused with febrile convulsions, when children have convulsions because of a high temperature (see page 21). Diarrhoea and vomiting may also trigger seizures because they can prevent the absorption of anti-epileptic drugs. Feeling generally poorly, or having a cold, may also make you more prone to seizures as your general resistance is lowered.

Excess alcohol

Too much alcohol is a common factor in seizures, though this does vary, as everyone's capacity is different. Anti-epileptic drugs may mean you have increased sensitivity to alcohol. Medical research suggests that drinking more than two units of alcohol in less than twelve to fifteen hours significantly increases the risk of seizures in people with epilepsy. (A unit of alcohol is a half-pint of beer or cider, a glass of wine or one measure – 'short' – of spirits such as whisky or gin.)

Heavy drinking tends also to be part of a package including late nights, missed meals and forgotten tablets, all of which may trigger seizures. Seizures also often occur as part of a hangover. Repeated heavy drinking can actually cause seizures in people without epilepsy. Around 20 per cent of alcoholic men and 10 per cent of alcoholic women develop major seizures, especially between the ages of forty-five and fifty.

One particular risk appears to relate to beer or cider drinking. This means swallowing a lot of fluid, and there is some evidence that too much fluid can in some cases cause seizures. Water intoxication has been mentioned as a particular feature of taking carbamazepine (Tegretol) – people taking this may find that their bodies may not be able to dispose of large quantities of fluid.

Drugs
Some drugs are known to lower seizure threshold. Apart from 'recreational' drugs, these include tricyclic anti-depressants, phenothiazines (for psychosis and severe nausea), isoniazid (used for TB) and high doses of penicillin. Certain other drugs interact with anti-epileptic medication, so always remind a new or visiting doctor that you have epilepsy if accepting a prescription.

Food
Some people have found that certain foods seem to make them more prone to seizures. Interestingly, given the link between epilepsy and migraine, these are often migraine triggers too – one woman, for example, reported that cheese, seafood, wine and chocolate seemed to set off attacks. Other substances have also been identified as possible triggers – for example, research from the University of Arizona linked the artifical sweetener aspartame with seizures. For more on food allergy and intolerance, see pages 78–9.

Perhaps most importantly, the majority of people with epilepsy have low blood sugar at the time of a seizure. Keeping to a regular food intake may therefore be key in preventing seizures, and this is looked at again on pages 71–4.

Nutrient shortages
Certain nutrient shortages have been linked with epilepsy and seizures – either through dietary deficiencies, or because the person's body is unable to absorb them from food because of a condition such as coeliac disease. Some anti-epileptic drugs deplete nutrients too (so does

stress). Shortages of vitamin B6 and D, and lack of essential minerals such as calcium and iron, have been blamed for triggering seizures. For more on how to correct possible nutritional deficiencies, see pages 74–7.

Menstruation and seizures

Some women find that they tend to have more seizures just before or during their period. It isn't really known why this happens, though some doctors believe it may be caused by alteration in hormonal levels of oestrogen and progesterone. It's possible that it is due to a combination of this and other factors such as increased fluid retention and changes in the blood levels of anti-epileptic medications. See page 72 for diet advice which might help with your hormones.

Mood

Sometimes certain moods seem to precede a seizure. These are often 'stereotyped' in that they follow the same sequence of events or feelings – a typical example could be a feeling of sullen depression, though occasionally some report elation instead. This may be called the 'prodromata' or events leading up to a seizure, and many doctors see this as coming from abnormal brain activity which finally builds up to an actual seizure. Partners or parents of those with epilepsy can often tell when a seizure is pending in their loved ones. However, another possibility is that the mood changes themselves cause the seizure.

Temperature

Sudden extreme changes in temperature have been cited as triggers for some, for example when the weather becomes very warm or rooms are overheated. In some unusually hot summers in the UK recently, there was a dramatic rise in seizures, for reasons not fully understood. Some people also report having more seizures in thundery weather because of the increased electrical activity, although this could also have a psychological component, in that some people find storms frightening and this fear in itself may be enough to increase the likelihood of seizures.

Flashing lights, TV, patterns and sounds

These are grouped together because they all relate to what is known as 'reflex' epilepsy, when people react to specific stimulus with a seizure.

Although the popular imagination has been caught by the image of flashing lights triggering seizures, only about 4 per cent of people have *photosensitive epilepsy*, in which seizures can be provoked by sensory stimulus such as flickering sunlight, strobe lights, television, videos and computers. The main dangers are from strobe lights flashing at a frequency of 15–60 flashes a second (ordinary disco lights often flash much slower than this) and most people have to be exposed to the stimulus for quite a time before it triggers a seizure. Television is probably more common than lights as a trigger, though of course you can have both – in America, there is a campaigning epilepsy group trying to have strobe-type lights banned from TV commercials.

A very few people seem to be acutely pattern-sensitive, and may have seizures triggered by, for example, horizontal lines, stripes as in a venetian blind, grids, weaves on clothing or squared patterns on linoleum.

A few people also may find their seizures are triggered by sudden loud noises, or by certain specific sounds such as trains or traffic. In the same way, a sudden shock or startle may act as a trigger.

Unique triggers

These can be highly idiosyncratic. Some people react to certain specific songs or colours; or may find their seizures triggered by smells such as glue, or sounds such as the telephone ringing or a siren. These probably belong among the reflex epilepsy triggers just covered, but because they are so individual they may well have a psychological component too – that is, at some point a person has learned to make an association between a certain stimulus and a seizure.

Checklist: seizure triggers

Common
Stress
Emotional upset
Lack of sleep
Excess alcohol
Infections and illnesses
Allergies
Pre-menstrual syndrome

Less common
Changes in temperature (especially sudden heat and including hot showers)
Particular smells
Certain sounds, such as music, traffic, drilling, sirens
Seeing patterns (some people are even sensitive to reading)
Flashing lights

Individual triggers – add your own

CHAPTER 4

How to help yourself

As a young man, Jack, receiving a diagnosis of epilepsy, also received a long list of 'don'ts' from his family doctor. Parties, late nights, too much exertion – he was warned that several aspects of living could trigger off a seizure. 'Well, that's the end of my life,' was his initial reaction.

Certainly, many family doctors will hand out 'received wisdoms' – standard common sense about epilepsy management such as making sure you get enough sleep and don't drink too much. Lifestyle management *is* important, as a third of all people with epilepsy find they have more seizures in times of stress. People with epilepsy generally seem to do better when hours and meals are regular, with enough sleep, proper diet and exercise.

But epilepsy is only ever part of someone's life, and it is possible to take an active part in treating your epilepsy, even if you cannot cure it. This means finding a balance that's right for you between taking risks in order to have a life, and avoiding seizures – generally, taking an active rather than a passive role.

Empowering yourself as far as possible is all the more important because epilepsy can affect so many other aspects of lifestyle. Taking responsibility for lifestyle issues is a vital step towards better health for many people with epilepsy.

Become informed about epilepsy
Learning about your type of epilepsy and seizures is one of the most important empowering steps you can take.

Being informed about epilepsy lessens stress, uncertainty and anxiety, and boosts self-esteem. Much can be done by informing yourself about epilepsy via books and epilepsy support groups. 'Well-informed patients make sure their doctors are well-informed,' as the Epilepsy Federation of America puts it.

You do need your family doctor and your epilepsy specialist in order to learn what type of epilepsy you have, and what treatment you individually need. Epilepsy organizations, though invaluable, cannot answer medical questions about your own particular condition. But many people find it difficult to obtain information about their own epilepsy. When a diagnosis is first made, they may be too shocked to ask the proper questions, or to absorb the information that is given. Or maybe their doctors seem too busy to answer questions. But it is your basic right to ask questions and receive answers. Common questions include:

- Exactly what type of epilepsy do I have?
- What other medications can I take?
- When do I take my tablets?
- What happens if I miss a dose?
- Can I drink?
- What might trigger a seizure?
- Do I need to consider other lifestyle issues such as stress?
- Could I have information about counselling to discuss new lifestyle issues which have arisen, such as a new relationship or bereavement?
- What about pregnancy and breastfeeding?
- Can I drive?
- Can I think about decreasing my medication?
- What should I do if I need to discuss my treatment between appointments?

Writing down questions and answers may be helpful. (See pages 46–56 for more on treatments available from your doctor.)

Relationships and emotions

Relationships can be a prime source of stress, which affects seizure patterns in many (see pages 28 and 81–85.) Although it doesn't happen to everyone, strong emotions can be enough to tip the balance and cause a seizure, especially if accompanied by other factors such as lack of sleep. 'Since we know from studies of animal species who have epilepsy that epilepsy is very much bound up with the emotions and fear and the "flight or fight" response, this connection with emotion is quite understandable and is sometimes a key to helping patients control their seizures, or avoid situations where seizures are most likely to occur,' says Dr Tim Betts, consultant in neuropsychiatry at the University of Birmingham in the UK. Some people with epilepsy may have fewer relationships. They may feel isolated by their condition, or be afraid – often without cause – that trust and friendship will be withdrawn once outsiders find out about their epilepsy. Telling others about epilepsy is a highly personal choice. Ideally, perhaps, it comes after a period in which the other has had the chance to get to know and appreciate you as a person. In this case, it may increase closeness, or add another whole new dimension to the relationship. It is certainly educational. Indeed, some individuals make a point of being open about epilepsy for this very reason.

Epilepsy itself can cause stress in a relationship. For example, many individuals have severe mood swings such as depression before and/or after seizures of which they themselves may not be aware, though their close ones may be. This *isn't* to say that all people with epilepsy are difficult to live with – just that epilepsy may, in some cases, bring its own specific problems. Mood swings are often thought to be caused by electrical activity in the brain which may lead up to a seizure (and an EEG would probably show this); depression, too, is a very natural reaction to having a seizure. Medication may also cause problem moods in some, such as irritability. There may also be specific psychological problems, such as fear of having a seizure when going out, which constricts a couple's or family's social life; or dependency on close people, for example with partners acting as substitute parents.

All in all, understanding and working on relationships can be very beneficial in reducing emotional stress, and so having a favourable effect on seizures. Discussion with your close others, keeping a diary and counselling are just some of the ways in which people make relationships more comprehensible and manageable.

Sexual difficulties are so common that it can be hard to say whether they are due to epilepsy, or the 'normal' problems with personal relationships which we may all have. This said, people with epilepsy may sometimes experience sexual difficulties because of seizures or drug treatment. This seems to be particularly true of people who have temporal lobe epilepsy. A change of drug, complementary therapies, or in some cases counselling may help. In the first instance ask your GP, who can refer you to more specialist services.

One particular concern expressed by some is fear of having a seizure during sexual activity, especially given the presumption that orgasm involves some form of 'paroxysmal discharge' within the brain, as neurologists Anthony Hopkins and Richard Appleton put it in their book on epilepsy (see page 120.) However, this is actually exceptionally rare, and possibly one of the least harmful environments in which to have a seizure anyway.

Identifying triggers
Everyone's epilepsy is different, so it can be helpful to see if you can identify what triggers seizures in your case (see pages 28–33 for more on seizure triggers).

Keeping a good, detailed seizure diary for at least three months is something many people find helpful, with details of activities, food and drink, social life, bedtimes, sleep, exercise and – often key – your feelings.

Mind, body and soul

Our spiritual awareness has an important bearing on our everyday health, so cultivating awareness of our psychic health in its widest perspective is key. Some people are acutely aware of their spiritual needs and may for example start feeling emotionally unbalanced, cranky or starved in some way if deprived of time for solitude and reflection. Others require a more structured approach in the form of a regular commitment to a spiritually oriented organization. Certainly, the links between psychic and bodily health are becoming more accepted even among conventional practitioners, and maintaining an awareness of this holistic approach can be seen as part of a person's individual responsibility for health. Mental, emotional and spiritual factors blend to influence physical health, as seen both from the conventional and from the complementary view. For example, you will derive more benefit from a regular drug regime or a soothing massage if you can at the same time manage to forgive someone whom you perceive as having intruded on you or offended you.

Some people have found it frustrating that, after keeping a seizure diary for months, they can't seem to find any link between external events and seizures. It may help to discuss your diary with another person to see if they can spot anything you've missed. However, for some people it is a fact of life that there doesn't seem to be any apparent link between outside factors and seizures.

Time management in general is something many people with epilepsy find helpful, as poor memory is common. Things which have worked well for some people include:

- Using lists
- Making notes
- Keeping a diary
- Taking time for yourself.

These may all seem very obvious, but are easily over-looked!

Enjoying life

'Sensible restrictions' are usually advised in certain activities, such as cycling and swimming, though everyone has to decide for him or herself which level of activity suits best. Jack, aged thirty-four, with fully controlled epilepsy, happily worked as a roofer, cycling to and from work each day. However, he steadily refused to swim, claiming he didn't feel safe in the water! Incidentally, research shows that few seizures happen in the water, perhaps because people are less likely to have them when enjoying themselves, though people with less well controlled epilepsy are usually advised to swim with a friend.

Many people refuse to let epilepsy dictate a way of life to them and, generally, there are very few activities which are absolutely forbidden, though you may well be advised to go with a friend and to take certain pre-cautions if you're planning some activities – for example, if rock-climbing, avoid being the leader, and ensure you are clipped in between other people. In the same way, you have to decide which of the basic safety precautions advocated you want to adopt at home.

Diet

From Hippocrates' time onwards, epilepsy has been treated with a wide range of special diets, vinegar and honey being a particular favourite of the ancients. Diet can indeed be a key factor in how well epilepsy is managed, and there's more on nutritional therapy on pages 71–80. Meanwhile, though, the rules for a good diet for anyone are simple:

- Eat a wide variety of foods.
- Include plenty of fresh fruit and vegetables.
- Avoid too much sugar and fat.

- Avoid processed foods when possible.
- Eat whole foods such as brown rice and wholemeal bread.
- Eat regularly – many people have low blood sugar at the time of a seizure. This applies particularly to busy people, and especially to mothers of young children.
- Some people with epilepsy have found that particular foods seem to trigger seizures, so some foods may be best avoided. Common allergens include wheat products, dairy products, chocolate, eggs, coffee, oranges, strawberries, additives, yeast and sugar.

Social drinking

For most people with epilepsy, the occasional drink over a meal or with friends isn't a problem (but see pages 29–30), though you may want to double-check with your doctor if you can safely drink on your current anti-epileptic medication. If you do take the occasional drink:

- Moderate wine drinking may be better than beer or cider if you are taking carbamazepine (because of the dangers of too much fluid).
- If you tend to do a lot of pub drinking where you and your friends buy in rounds, and feel you want to stick to your limits without spoiling the fun, try and opt for half-pints instead of pints, or alternate beer with shandy (i.e. a small amount of beer mixed with lemonade). Low-alcohol or non-alcoholic beer is another option.
- Make sure you also take your medication.
- The occasional late night will do no harm, but don't let regular drinking make you miss too much sleep, or meals.
- If you have a hangover, try to lie in, take some vitamin C, have something to eat and generally take it easy – many seizures take place after the drinking, not during it.

Seizure alert dogs

Dogs' acute sensitivity to various phenomena is well known, including their awareness of their owners' moods and emotions, and their sensing of impending changes in the weather, particularly thunderstorms. Some people in the UK and the USA have 'seizure alert dogs' which have been trained to alert their owners when a seizure is imminent.

There are differing theories as to how the dogs work. One is that they work by smell – that a seizure is preceded by a chemical change somewhere in the body, which the dog can detect. Another theory relates to electromagnetic field changes. Every body is surrounded by an electromagnetic field, and some believe that this field becomes disrupted before a seizure and that a dog can detect this. It may also be that subtle changes in behaviour and mood can be picked up by the dog before they become apparent to people around or the individual concerned. There is also an unmeasured but valuable effect – because the person knows he or she can trust the dog, he or she is likely to be more relaxed, which in itself may reduce seizure activity.

Most breeds can act as seizure alert dogs, but, as the bond of trust between dog and owner is vital, most of the dogs are (or become) the owner's pet. Before being trained, the dog has a full examination to make sure it is physically and mentally capable of doing the work. The dog is then trained with its owner, which may take less or more time depending on how quickly the dog gets the idea. In the UK, at Support Dogs in Sheffield, advanced training is followed up with video monitoring at home and final assessments before the dog is given Seizure Alert Dog status. Each dog is taught tasks specific for its owner's needs, and to respond to the person's specific type of seizure activity. The dogs cost around £1,500 to train but no charge is made to the person with epilepsy – Support Dogs is a charity dependent on contributions and outside funding.

An animal who gets the idea of working as a seizure alert dog can be remarkably accurate. The exception may be with seizures caused by strobe lights, perhaps because they come on too quickly for the dog to pick up any prior warning.

Case history: Seizure alert dogs

Anna-Maria, aged twenty-eight, is a make-up artist living in the USA who owns a seizure alert dog, Barret, a red setter. Anna-Maria suffers complex partial attacks with an aura which begins with stomach churning and then proceeds to hearing far-off bells and strange voices. 'Barret has always seemed to know when a seizure was imminent and would follow me round or come and find me if we weren't in the same room. When a seizure is imminent, he acts distressed, puts his tail between his legs, and pins his ears back, whining. Then he begins pawing at me, pulling at me and making me lie down.'

Anna-Maria's attacks are controlled by medication for around three-quarters of the time, but her remaining seizures are highly unpredictable. She tried keeping a seizure diary and couldn't find any links between her activities, emotions and seizures. As her work requires a steady hand and quite a bit of concentration, she does need the peace of mind a reliable dog can give, so she can attend to her clients with complete confidence. 'My dog has always been 100 per cent accurate – I didn't believe it when first told of the idea, but I've seen him in action too many times to doubt now.'

Stigma

Just a few years ago, in 1995, a woman with epilepsy, who was having counselling in order to improve her confidence, had the misfortune to have a seizure in a public store. She came round to find herself surrounded by members of the public gawping, while in a corner one woman was saying to another, 'They say they're possessed by the devil, you know.' More work for the counsellor!

This story illustrates all too clearly that, owing to ignorance about epilepsy, stigma can still be a problem. The stupidity of the comment above must be rare, but does represent the extreme end of public uneasiness about epilepsy. Surveys show that attitudes are changing slowly, and that fear of stigma itself may be worse than the actual thing, but the fact remains that some people will be unfortunate in the attitudes to epilepsy they come across.

'I'm quite open about my epilepsy and tend to tell people because I think it helps people be informed about epilepsy. I did lose a few people I thought were friends when I first told people – but I tell myself that they can't really have been true friends, can they?' – Emma

'I'm not interested in announcing to the world that I've got epilepsy. If people look like being friends, or there's a special reason, like a job, then I might talk about it. I just want to take my medication and get on with my life.' – Jack

Being open about epilepsy is educational for the general public, but to act as an ambassador for epilepsy is not what some people want, preferring to guard their privacy and dignity. What is perhaps more important to individual health is fear of stigma, which may create lack of confidence which in turn can affect well-being, lifestyle and general health. Your individual fears, and individual attitudes to epilepsy, can affect your self-esteem, and may need to be tackled before you try to change other people's approaches. For some, this may mean counselling, and there's more on this on page 94.

What to do in the event of a seizure
Attacks cannot be stopped, so advice from the National Society for Epilepsy in the UK suggests the following guidelines:

Boosting personal awareness and self-esteem
Confidence-boosting measures recommended by the
British Epilepsy Association include:

- Going for what you want and refusing to use epilepsy as
  an excuse if life doesn't turn out as you wish.
- Focusing on the positive aspects of having epilepsy (e.g.
  you may take more care of your health, diet and fitness).
- Being assertive – everyone needs to do this at times but
  it may have more relevance than usual for people with
  epilepsy, who are at particular risk of low self-esteem.

During a convulsive seizure
At the start of the attack the person may cry out as air
is expelled through the voice box, breathing may stop
and the person may go slightly blue. Frightening though
this looks, it is normal, and the person is not in pain and
will have little or no memory of the event.

- Prevent others from crowding round.
- Put something soft under the person's head (like a
  jacket). Only move the person if he or she is in danger
  (e.g. in the road).
- Do not try to restrain the person's convulsive
  movements.
- Do not put anything in the person's mouth as the
  teeth can easily be broken. (There is no danger of
  the tongue being swallowed.)

Once the convulsions have stopped
- Roll the person on to their side to the recovery
  position.
- Wipe away any excess saliva and, if breathing is still
  laboured, check that nothing is blocking the throat
  such as dentures or food.
- Do all you can to minimize any embarrassment. If the

person has been incontinent, deal with this as quickly as possible.
- Stay with the person, giving reassurance until he or she has fully recovered.

Non-convulsive seizures
- Gently guide them away from obvious dangers like wandering into the road.
- Prevent others from crowding around.
- Stay with the person until he or she has recovered. Bear in mind that he or she may be confused.

Get medical help: if a seizure lasts longer than five minutes; is immediately followed by another; if the person has badly injured him or herself during the seizure; or has trouble breathing after the seizure.

CHAPTER 5

Conventional treatments

There is one main choice from conventional medicine when it comes to treating epilepsy – drugs, which achieve seizure control in 70–80 per cent of people. After a lull of several years, there are now new anti-epileptic drugs on the market. Surgery is another option, but it is rarely prescribed. With recent and pending drug developments, people with epilepsy may find they have more choice than before. However, the problems of side-effects remain for many.

Diagnosing epilepsy

A diagnosis of epilepsy is a serious matter, and not one your doctor will make lightly. Apart from the medical implications, it affects education, work, leisure, insurance, driving and many other aspects of lifestyle.

Also, diagnosing epilepsy is not always straightforward. There can be many reasons for loss of consciousness, and your doctor may need to make further investigations to make sure that you are not suffering from some other disorder.

A detailed medical history is particularly important, as other diagnostic methods such as EEG (see below) may not always be able to record an actual seizure. Your doctor will ask you about the pattern of any past seizures, and may ask whether you had birth complications or head injuries. The doctor may also ask you certain questions, such as:

- Did you have any warning (aura) before the attack,

such as a churning feeling in the stomach, or a feeling of fear?
- What were you doing at the time of the attack?
- Were you hungry, thirsty, hot or tired?
- Were you undergoing any severe stress or feeling any strong emotion such as anger or excitement?
- Did you feel unwell, for example, sick or dizzy?
- Exactly what can you remember of the attack and how long did it seem to last?
- When you came round, what was your first memory and how did you feel, physically (weak, shaky) and emotionally (confused, weepy)?

Sometimes it is useful for a partner or friend to help answer these questions, as most people retain no memory of the seizure, and may be confused about its start and its aftermath.

Diagnostic techniques
Specialist techniques are available to help your doctor decide whether you have epilepsy.

Electroencephalogram (EEG)
This test measures the electrical activity of your brain cells, using several electrodes which are placed on the head. A printout is produced of your brain waves to see if they show epileptic patterns, though some EEGs appear normal between seizures. To obtain a more consistent result, your doctor may also want to you to have:

EEG ambulatory monitoring: This allows the brain's electrical patterns to be recorded over several hours, while you carry on with normal activities. EEG electrodes are attached to the scalp as before, but connect to a small portable tape recorder which records your brain waves.

Video telemetry: Available at some hospitals, video telemetry is when both EEG and video recordings are made to try to record a seizure on video. Electrodes are attached to the scalp, and the person can usually move freely round the room.

Brain scan

Depending on the results of the EEG, your doctor may refer you for a brain scan, which looks for any structural damage within the brain (scars, growths) which could be causing seizures.

Computerized tomography (CT or CAT): The most common type of brain scan, CT (computed tomography) involves taking X-rays of the brain which are then visualized by means of a computer. Several tiny narrow beams of radiation pass through the brain from different angles, providing a cross-section of pictures in 'slices'. These pictures are then analysed by computer, and may show the more obvious sort of damage or abnormality.

Magnetic resonance imaging (MRI): This is a scanning technique which bounces magnetic fields and radio waves off the brain to form very detailed pictures of the brain structure. The MR machine detects radio signals from the hydrogen atoms in the brain and creates a picture based on these signals. This gives a much more precise view of subtle abnormalities, such as small tumours or minor developmental abnormalities, and can help determine treatment.

MRI spectroscopy: A refinement of MRI, this measures metabolites, chemicals within the brain. This gives information about normal and abnormal brain cells, and might also be used to pinpoint the site of lesions before neurosurgery.

Positron emission tomography (PET): In a few research centres, positron emission tomography imaging is used to identify areas of the brain which are producing seizures. It measures the metabolic activity of the brain. A small amount of radioactive material (isotopes) is injected into a vein in the arm, and this concentrates in certain areas, such as tumours, and makes the image stronger.

Blood tests

Blood tests are done to check your overall health and to test for any underlying condition which could be causing seizures. (They can also be used to monitor levels of anti-epileptic drugs – see **Drug monitoring,** below.)

Treatment/anti-epileptic drugs

The aim of anti-epileptic drugs is to control your seizures without side-effects. If this is not possible, a compromise goal is to reduce the frequency or intensity of seizures with the fewest possible side-effects.

Drugs don't treat epilepsy itself – that is, they don't usually eliminate the causes of epilepsy (unless this is a separate disease). They prevent seizures by reducing the amount of electrical activity in the brain. In other words, they suppress the symptoms of epilepsy, but don't treat the underlying problem – this remains a goal for future research.

There was a lull of over twenty years in the development of anti-epileptic drugs but the scene has changed dramatically in the last few years. Newer drugs introduced in the UK are vigabatrin, lamotrigine, piracetam, gabapentin and topiramate (generic or international names). Zonizimide has also been licensed in Japan and felbamate in the United States. New drugs are also under development, including remacemide, tiagabine and levetiracetam.

The chart on page 50 lists some common epilepsy drugs and side-effects, but is by no means exhaustive. Read the product information sheet that accompanies drugs, or ask your doctor or pharmacist for more information.

Drug monitoring

Drugs are usually started at a low dose which is then built up until seizure control is achieved. Drugs won't work properly until they reach a certain level in the body, and that level has to be maintained. It is important

Established drugs		
Drug name (generic)	**Useful for**	**Common side-effects**
Carbamazepine	Partial, generalized tonic-clonic	Drowsiness, skin rash
Sodium valproate	Generalized tonic-clonic, juvenile myoclonic, partial, absences and other generalized	Tremor, weight gain, hair loss (reversible), liver damage (extremely rare)
Phenytoin	Partial, generalized tonic-clonic	Drowsiness, acne, gum overgrowth, coarsening of facial features with prolonged use
Newer drugs		
Vigabatrin	Partial	Drowsiness, stomach complaints, headache, occasional depression
Gabapentin	Partial, secondarily generalized	Drowsiness, fatigue weight gain, dizziness
Lamotrigine	Partial, secondarily generalized tonic-clonic	Skin rashes (very occasionally dangerous), headache, drowsiness

to follow your doctor's instructions very carefully as to when and how much medication should be taken.

Your doctor will use blood tests to help achieve the right dosage of the drug. Drugs are absorbed into the bloodstream and from there pass to the brain, where they achieve their effect.

If the initial dose doesn't help, your doctor might suggest trying a higher dose. If that still doesn't work, your doctor may withdraw the first drug and try a second one. Doctors prefer to use just one drug if possible (monotherapy) but if seizures are not controlled, they may try more a combination of drugs (polytherapy).

Case history: Emma

Emma Shand's first seizure was brought to her attention in dramatic circumstances at the age of nineteen – she crashed her car because of it. Luckily, the accident was not serious and her family and friends were very supportive. After a second seizure, Emma was put on carbamazepine. An initial side-effect was sleepiness, so the dose was adjusted so that Emma took the larger part of her drugs in the evening. After a while, Emma felt she might be able to manage on a lower dose and requested another blood test from her doctor in order to see if this was possible. Her dose was successfully lowered, and she now takes one and a half instead of two tablets a day.

Emma, now twenty-six, leads a busy life as a marketing executive, in which epilepsy does not really interfere. 'Obviously, I know my limits and stick to them, but I do go out, have the odd social drink with my friends, and generally enjoy life. I try to be as positive as possible about having epilepsy and see myself as lucky in that it doesn't affect me too much, and that I've found a manageable drug regime. Epilepsy has also made me aware that life isn't all roses, and that illness is a reality for many people.'

Taking your prescribed drugs

Taking your drugs as prescribed is one of the most important factors in maintaining seizure control. Medical research shows that, left untreated over a long period, epileptic seizures can lead to further neurological damage – in other words, untreated epilepsy is progressive, and can be harmful. However, some people feel their medication is inappropriate, and may often feel over-medicated, especially if they have only had a couple of minor seizures in childhood. If you are unhappy about your drug regime, make an appointment with your doctor specifically to discuss this.

Side-effects
Were it not for anti-epileptic drugs, many people with epilepsy would not be able to lead a normal life. But there are side-effects. These include drowsiness, inability to concentrate and memory problems. Other side-effects include bone softening, reduced production of red blood cells, swelling of the gums, emotional disturbances and loss of motor co-ordination. There can be cosmetic side-effects, too, such as extra hair growth on the face and yellowing of the skin.

Side-effects can be a sign that the dose you are on is too high, or has been increased too rapidly. Side-effects do sometimes pass off as the body becomes accustomed to the drug, but if not, tell your doctor, who may try a lower dose or, later, a second drug.

The question of side-effects is something you and your doctor need to discuss in the context of quality of life. Building up a dose gradually, and giving the body time to adjust, may help. Taking a calculated risk with a drug may be worth it if it achieves control of seizures which happen several times a week; but you may not feel it is worth undergoing side-effects if you have seizures three or four times a year.

Giving up or reducing your drugs
There is a case for coming off medication if you have been seizure-free for two years. Some studies show that 50–60 per cent of people who remain free of seizures can eventually stop taking medication without the seizures coming back. And a study by the Medical Research Council in the UK showed that two-thirds of patients remained seizure-free after being weaned off drugs.

Unfortunately, there is no way of predicting whether seizures will return or not in any particular person, though the Medical Research Council's study indicated that those who did worst were patients taking more than one anti-epileptic drug, or with a history of neonatal seizures. In practice many patients and doctors are wary of giving up drugs because of the practical as well as health implications (e.g. jobs, insurance, driving licence). Drug reduction should take place only under competent medical supervision.

Surgery

Surgery involves removing the tiny section of brain tissue responsible for seizures. It has been estimated that surgery could help around a third of people with diffi-cult-to-treat epilepsy where only a part of the brain is affected (mostly the temporal lobe). While many doctors believe that more routine referral for surgery would be helpful, in practice surgery is usually only prescribed as a last resort. Just 1,500 operations are performed for epilepsy each year in the United States. Also, there are very stringent medical and psychological tests to make sure that the benefits would outweigh the risks of brain surgery.

Today, surgery is a relatively safe and sophisticated option thanks to advanced scanning techniques like MRI, and to new surgical techniques, such as 'multiple subpial transection', which can be used to avoid interfering with important areas of the brain, for example those governing movement or speech. It involves cutting the cortex into tiny slices in such a way as to stop epileptic activity moving across them, while leaving the essential nerve connections intact.

It is estimated that around 65 per cent of patients become seizure-free after surgery, or only experience mild auras, while 85 per cent enjoy enough benefit to make the operation justifiable. Severe complications occur in fewer than 5 per cent of cases. The risks are the same as any other major neurosurgical operation, with up to a 1 per cent mortality rate. There is also a slight risk of stroke (2 per cent) and of developing eye problems (2 per cent).

However, many people naturally have doubts at the thought of brain surgery, no matter how minute and specialized. Some people have reported severe headaches and general feelings of illness for a while after surgery. Also, there are not many centres where surgery can be performed, so waiting lists are long.

Vagal nerve stimulation

A small device similar to a pacemaker is inserted into the body so that it vibrates against the vagus nerve, which is connected to the parts of the brain thought to produce seizures. Stimulation of the vagus nerve may disrupt the abnormal electrical activity in the brain that causes seizures.

VNS is still experimental, not widely available, and only a few of those treated have achieved a significant lessening of seizures. Long-term side-effects have not been established as this treatment is so new. In the short term, some people have reported pain in the throat, ear or tooth, which can be lessened if the doctor adjusts the generator's programming. Some have also complained of nausea. VNS is also being used in the USA, where it is known as NeuroCybernetic Prosthesis (NCP®) System.

To treat or not to treat

This isn't as easy a decision as it might seem. There is evidence to show that starting treatment earlier rather than later helps prevent epilepsy getting worse. However, some recent research shows that untreated epilepsy seems to clear up of its own accord in some people. One Dutch study of over 200 children delayed treatment until they had had four seizures, and found that 40 per cent of them became seizure-free without drugs. However, bear in mind that 70–80 per cent of people do become seizure-free with the right drug, and that the best treatment is the one which you and your doctor decide on together.

Women and epilepsy

There are certain special situations associated with women and epilepsy. Your doctor may suggest dealing with seizures around menstruation (so-called 'catamenial epilepsy') by prescribing a diuretic to reduce water retention; increasing your usual dose of anti-epileptic medication just before a period; taking the contraceptive pill and progesterone therapy; or prescribing drugs such as clobazam, an 'add-on' anti-epileptic drug.

Contraception is another issue. Some anti-epileptic medications – carbamazepine, phenytoin and phenobarbitone – interact with the contraceptive pill, making it less reliable, so again this may need to be discussed with your doctor.

Women with epilepsy who are planning to become pregnant should talk to their doctors before conceiving, or as early in pregnancy as possible. The vast majority of women with epilepsy have normal pregnancies which result in healthy babies; however, some anti-epileptic drugs do increase the risk of abnormalities such as cleft palate, so your doctor may need to withdraw or change drugs for pregnancy.

Pregnancy itself sometimes triggers changes in seizure patterns, though this varies. Some women report that seizures are more frequent, though in an estimated 50 per cent of cases epilepsy is better controlled during pregnancy, perhaps because they are more careful about getting enough sleep and taking medication regularly. The available evidence suggests that women with frequent seizures unfortunately tend to find they happen even more frequently; and women carrying a boy may for reasons yet unknown also have more frequent seizures. Most women with epilepsy have normal deliveries – in labour, only 1–2 per cent of women with active epilepsy will have a tonic-clonic seizure.

Generally, breastfeeding is possible for women with epilepsy, as even if you are taking medication, only small amounts pass through to the baby, who has in any case been exposed to medication while in the womb. Lack of sleep may take on particular meaning for new mothers with epilepsy – do enlist your doctor's support in planning a routine for your baby which allows you as much rest as possible, for example introducing a bottle so that someone else can give night feeds.

CHAPTER 6

The natural therapies and epilepsy

From the time of the ancient Greeks onwards, natural therapies for epilepsy have abounded. And in the last ten years there has been an explosion of interest in complementary therapies as more and more people, dissatisfied with the limits of conventional medicine, are taking their health and their lives into their own hands.

This was acknowledged by the medical establishment in a landmark report by the British Medical Association (BMA) in 1993. This report conceded for the first time not only that natural therapies are here to stay but also that some of them should, and probably would, become more available to everyone.

This change in thinking is slowly filtering through the conventional medical establishment. Many doctors who deal with people with epilepsy are coming to realize the value of treating the whole person, rather than simply suppressing the symptoms with drugs. Today there is much emphasis on quality of life, as well as seizure control.

The return of traditional medicine has resulted in a host of new ideas entering the already wide menu of therapies. But what exactly are these therapies and how do they differ from the conventional medical approach? Why do people go to natural therapists? Above all, could a natural therapist help you manage your epilepsy and, if so, how can you find a trustworthy therapist? The remainder of this book sets out to make that choice a lot clearer and easier.

Why go to a natural therapist?

A natural therapist is, or should be, someone who not only understands you and your condition, but is also familiar with safe and gentle treatments that do not involve you being filled with drugs or operated on.

People often turn to a natural therapist when they've explored all other avenues and feel that 'it can't make it any worse'. Perhaps they're sick of having tried every drug on the market without success and still having continuing seizures – this happens in some 20–30 per cent of cases. Or they may feel that owing to the side-effects of drugs, they're not living life to the full – sadly, side-effects have been described as 'a way of life' for many people with epilepsy. Or maybe it's a case of wanting to improve general well-being and health, or to tackle other accompanying complaints, for example depression or migraine, both of which are common in people with epilepsy.

Whatever the reasons people go to natural practitioners, they often seem to get a high level of satisfaction. In Britain, for example, where no therapist is legally required to train to practise non-medical therapy, surveys in recent years have consistently shown satisfaction levels between 60 and 80 per cent.

Consulting your doctor or epilepsy specialist

This is very important in epilepsy. Achieving the right balance of drugs in your body can be a delicate and long-term process, and not one that a complementary practitioner should tinker with. Close liaison between conventional and alternative doctors is vital if you are thinking of decreasing medication. However, these days, conventional practitioners are more likely to be encouraging with regard to natural remedies for those with epilepsy. It's all part of the current climate in which people with epilepsy are being encouraged to take more of their health into their own hands. Also, very few complementary approaches will interfere with any drug treatment, but be cautious with herbs and aromatherapy (see pages 67–8). In the holistic concept, any forms of therapy can work together, including conventional ones. Complementary therapies can work to improve the many balances of the body towards a state of wellness. If the tendency of seizures diminishes under a broader programme, then an additional effect is that less anti-convulsant medication will be needed.

The principles behind natural therapies

There is quite a discussion (not to say argument, even among natural therapists themselves) about whether natural therapies operate under one guiding set of principles. The British Medical Association believes they do not – in a recent report, the BMA said that natural therapies were a mix of styles and techniques with nothing in common. That may be true superficially – applying an acupuncture needle is quite different to prescribing a vitamin supplement or giving a massage. But, underneath, the natural approaches do operate on certain common underlying principles:

- The body has a natural ability to heal itself and remain stable (homeostasis).
- People are not simply physical machines, like cars, but a subtle and complex blend of body, mind and emotions (or spirit or soul) all of which may play a part in health. In other words, an individual is not a collection of moving parts but a fully integrated whole. 'Holistic medicine' means treating this whole person – body, mind, emotions and spirit.
- Environmental and social conditions are just as important as a person's physical and psychological make-up and may have just as big an impact on health.

- Treating the root cause or causes of a problem is more important than treating the obvious immediate symptoms. Treating only symptoms may simply cover up the real underlying problem and make it worse, so that it reappears later as something more serious.
- Each person is an individual and cannot be treated in exactly the same way as anyone else.
- Healing is quicker and more effective if the person takes central responsibility for his or her own health and has an active involvement in the healing process (but a good therapist will also recognize when someone needs to 'let go' and place themselves in the hands of another).
- Good health is a state of emotional, mental, spiritual and physical 'balance'. Balance is fundamental to the concept of health in natural therapy. Ill health, say its exponents, is the result of being in a state of imbalance, or 'dis-ease'. The Chinese express this as the principle of yin and yang.
- There is a natural healing 'force' in the universe. The Chinese call this *qi* or *chi* (pronounced 'chee'), the Japanese *ki*, Indians *prana*. In the West it used to be called by its Latin name *vis medicatrix naturae*, or 'natural healing force', shortened today to 'life force'. A natural practitioner can help patients strengthen and balance this life energy, so helping them heal themselves.

How natural therapies differ

While natural therapies all share the same fundamental principles outlined above, they can be divided into two fairly distinct categories: physical therapies and psychological therapies.

For example, nutritional therapy and massage are obviously aimed at your body, while meditation and hypnotherapy target the mind. Often, there is a great overlap. Aromatherapy, for example, especially as used in epilepsy, treats both body and mind, and this kind of psychological training, which may involve some mental discipline, plays quite an important part in many complementary therapies for epilepsy.

Generally, improving your mental state will help improve your overall health as well, either by making you more relaxed, or because you become more positive and change aspects of your lifestyle and attitudes that were previously threatening your health.

In addition, some believe there is a third dimension to natural therapies. These are the so-called 'energy' therapies which often work on the idea of correcting the imbalances that cause 'dis-ease'. Energy therapies, such as acupuncture, work at restoring the body's natural energy or 'life force' at a subtle level.

This overall approach makes natural therapies ideal for epilepsy as it is a physical condition which can have strong emotional components. Any therapy which helps reduce stress – for example meditation and biofeedback – may be of real help in getting epilepsy more under control.

Natural therapies helpful for epilepsy

This is still a very new field and no one therapy will offer a magic cure for epilepsy. Often people have found that therapies, on their own or in combination, have worked as part of an overall self-help effort. In fact, the amount of effort you put in can be key in some of the therapies, especially the behavioural or psychological ones such as self-hypnosis.

Consulting your doctor or epilepsy specialist remains very important. However, these days many conventional practitioners are likely to be encouraging with regard to patients taking more responsibility for lifestyle management.

Pharmaceutical companies are actively exploring the ecology before our natural resources are wiped out, and are looking at cultures where age-old wisdoms about plant remedies have been handed down from generation to generation. In other words, conventional medicine is increasingly coming to recognize how much natural remedies have to offer. Some doctors do still have valid objections – for example that serious diseases may be missed or that a few practitioners advise patients to abandon orthodox treatment altogether. However, these objections can usually be overcome by making sure you attend faithfully all appointments with your own family doctor and epilepsy specialist, and stick closely to any treatment they have prescribed.

It can be very difficult to predict just which therapy will be beneficial, because epilepsy varies so widely in type and severity. People with epilepsy have been found to respond in very different ways to different therapies, but natural therapies which have been found helpful by some people with epilepsy include:

- Acupuncture (including acupressure and shiatsu)
- Alexander Technique
- Aromatherapy
- Biofeedback
- Chiropractic
- Counselling and psychotherapy
- Flower remedies
- Herbal remedies
- Homeopathy
- Hypnosis/self-hypnosis
- Massage
- Meditation
- Nutritional therapy
- Osteopathy
- Reflexology
- Traditional Chinese Herbal Medicine (TCHM)
- Yoga

How do natural remedies treat epilepsy?

One of the best things about natural remedies for epilepsy is that they can safely be used in conjunction with prescribed drugs. In some cases, a complementary therapy used together with prescribed medication may give the edge on seizure control. In other cases, people have been known to wean themselves off drugs with the help of natural remedies. Epilepsy is usually viewed as a dynamic, not a static disorder, which means that it can progress and change. In practice, this means that conventional drug doses may have to be reassessed anyway from time to time. In some cases, epilepsy gets better on its own after a period of years, and some people are able to give up their medication. All this gives more scope for natural remedies as forming part of a lifestyle which is as relaxed, balanced and seizure-free as possible.

Natural therapies may not be able to cure the underlying cause of your epilepsy. However, they will take into account any lifestyle issues which could impact on the frequency and severity of your seizures. This could include what you eat, how much exercise you take, smoking and drinking habits, how much stress you are under at work, and the state of your marriage or other close relationships.

Natural therapists may also view the frequency and severity of attacks as reflecting your internal state of health (psychological or physical) or energy balance, and may try to redress this as far as possible with a wide range of therapies. These therapies may work at avoiding psychological triggers of seizures such as emotional upset, perhaps by deep relaxing massage; or they may try to avoid allergens; or they may try to redress nutritional deficiencies. There's more information on exactly which therapies may help in the next three chapters.

A few people have found that certain natural remedies appear to make their epilepsy worse. For example, some people have reported that acupuncture and chiropractic have actually seemed to trigger seizures. Currently, there are no agreed protocols for treating people with epilepsy in either of these therapies. And, because to date there is so little organized research, such side-effects are anecdotal and could be random unlucky individual reactions. In other cases, it is definitely known that aspects of some treatments need to be avoided – for example, certain aromatherapy oils and even some supplements, such as evening primrose oil, have been shown to trigger seizures. In this case, these should definitely be avoided. Whatever therapy you feel drawn to, it is very important that you feel comfortable with your choice before continuing with it.

The significance of taking control

Taking control may have especially poignant significance for the person with epilepsy, at the mercy of a condition which 'seizes' them and flings them into a situation where they are completely out of control.

Epilepsy is often different from other disorders in that the person has very limited experience of the attacks, particularly if they are the sort which come on quickly and without warning. Once the seizure is over, the person may remember only the start, and have no memory of the actual attack itself. He or she is therefore dependent on others to assess their severity and to describe them. From this, it's an easy step to depending on others for treatment. Natural remedies give a chance to redress the balance, as it means taking treatment into your own hands.

This taking control has further relevance in the emotional aspects of epilepsy. As seizures for many are bound up with strong feelings, such as fear, anger and excitement, taking control of the emotions has obvious significance when it comes to treating epilepsy.

Most of all, it's a 'given' in any healing process that taking an active part in your own healing is an important factor in the success of many natural therapies. This is why a good practitioner will always encourage you to do this, even if it just means recommending a simple change in lifestyle.

Spiritual dimension to healing

Most family doctors believe that spirituality can help the healing process, according to an American survey. While traditional medications and surgery are still a necessary part of proper medical care, many recoveries can't be explained only in terms of medical procedures, the doctors surveyed agree.

The study showed that:

- Over 99 per cent of the doctors questioned believed that a person's spiritual attitude could contribute positively to the healing process.
- Another 80 per cent believed in the palliative powers of meditation and prayer.
- More than 55 per cent of the doctors surveyed said they use relaxation and meditation techniques in their practice.

Many of the doctors said they believed that healing takes place on a more subtle plane than the merely physical, and said they saw many weekly examples of mind/spirit healing.

The survey, done by a research company, formed part of a Spirituality and Healing in Medicine course run by the non-profit John Templeton Foundation, created in 1987 to examine the relationship between spirituality, morality and scientific method.

CHAPTER 7

Treating your body

Therapies which work on the body can improve physical confidence as well as overall health. Some therapies which work directly on your physical body have also been recommended for epilepsy either because they are relaxing and so reduce stress (such as massage), or because they may help treat the underlying cause of epilepsy (such as nutritional therapy). None claim to cure epilepsy – but all may improve it.

Cannabis – on prescription or a forbidden alternative?
The anti-convulsant properties of cannabis were investigated in the nineteenth century, and, as it has an analgesic effect, it was once widely used as a sedative or narcotic agent. More recently, its anti-convulsant and anti-spasmodic properties have been the subjects of scientific scrutiny again. A study by Dr J Cunha in 1980 looked at the effects of giving 200–300mg cannabidiol or placebo to sixteen drug-resistant patients, as well as their regular medication, and found that it did seem to have some beneficial effect. Of the patients who received the cannabis product:

- Three showed complete improvement.
- Two showed partial improvement.
- Two had minor improvement.
- One remained unchanged.
- And the only side-effect was mild sedation.

Of the patients who received the placebo:

- One improved.

- Seven remained unchanged.

Cannabis can now only be prescribed in the UK with special permission from the Home Secretary, and similar restrictions have applied in the USA since 1970; in 1996, fewer than ten people in the USA were legally allowed to use cannabis on medical grounds. Physicians risk being struck off if they prescribe cannabis illegally. Some individuals report weaning themselves off prescribed medicine and still being seizure-free if on cannabis – but often face legal problems and indeed imprisonment!

Many doctors believe it is only a matter of time before cannabis becomes more available. A survey by the British Medical Association News Review in the UK showed that nearly 80 per cent of hospital doctors believe cannabis should be available on a prescription-only basis for special therapeutic purposes in certain cases of neurological disease.

Herbal medicine

Herbal medicine, or phytotherapy as it is known in Europe, is the use of plants to heal. Many orthodox medicines are based on plant remedies – willow bark and aspirin is a well-known example. However, these should be used with caution in epilepsy – just because they are natural does not mean they are always safe. Do not buy over-the-counter remedies, and, as anyone can set up as a herbalist, check qualifications.

The popular herbal remedy St John's Wort, tradition-ally used for depression, could be a significant health risk for people already on medication, according to American research. Patients being treated for epilepsy, HIV or AIDS, on blood thinning medication, or who have had an organ transplant are at particular risk of a reaction if they also take the over-the-counter herb. Herbs said to be good for epilepsy include:

- Blue vervain, for absence seizures, especially if associated with seizures triggered by menstrual changes.
- Hyssop, which may be used in absence attacks.
- Lobelia, which is said to have a general depressant action on the central nervous system and so can be prescribed for epilepsy.
- Skullcap, which is supposed to relax states of nervous tension and the central nervous system.

A herbalist may create individual mixes of herbs depending on what sort of person you are, and whether you have any other existing health problems.

Massage
Research has shown that when elderly people lose a partner, one of the things they miss most is the closeness of touch. At the other end of the scale, babies fail to thrive without the warmth of close contact.

Massage can be very simple (and inexpensive) if you try it out at home, and can leave you wonderfully soothed and relaxed. Done professionally, it may have other characteristics, from a hefty kneading in order to unknot stiff joints, to a very gentle kind of 'laying on of hands' healing type of massage, like 'Therapeutic Touch'.

Naturopathy
Naturopathy is a truly holistic approach which involves treating a person with a mixture of different therapies.

Case history: Jessica

A naturopathic doctor in the USA helped nine-year-old Jessica, whose seizures dropped dramatically from one every three or four days to none at all. She started off with cranial osteopathy (or cranio-sacral treatments as they're known in the USA), and she found the very gentle head massage immensely relaxing. The naturopath also helped her parents, Al and Valerie, to make changes in her diet, including supplements of flax seed oil. 'We were amazed at how Jessica got her tonic-clonic seizures under control immediately with the treatment,' says Al Davidson. 'Two years on, Jessica has had no seizures and still has the occasional session of cranial osteopathy, but more because she enjoys it than to keep the epilepsy at bay. We also continue to pay close attention to her diet — she doesn't eat anything containing wheat, and takes a specially prescribed supplement every day.'

In epilepsy, a naturopath might look for nutritional imbalances, food allergies and intolerance, as well as considering psychological factors and exercises. Some naturopaths are qualified in other disciplines such as osteopathy and homeopathy, and many make use also of hydrotherapy, or water therapy, which ranges from salt baths to bathing in warm thermal springs.

Osteopathy/cranial osteopathy/chiropractic
Although osteopathy is usually thought of as a treatment for back problems, it can be used for a whole variety of musculoskeletal problems. Therapists say it aims to treat the whole person not just across the body, but across time, too, reaching right back to complications which might have been incurred during a difficult birth. Some osteopaths believe that every cell in the body records its autobiography, and that this 'cellular biology' becomes the body's biology

Osteopaths may use several techniques, such as massage, manipulation or stretching. In cranial osteopathy, they use very gentle manipulation to correct parts of the skull which may have been pushed out of place by traumatic birth or a car accident. Indeed, so gentle is cranial osteopathy that a therapist may seem to be doing no more than laying on hands, although in fact from this stance he or she will be looking at the person's body patterns, spine position, breathing and areas of the brain which link up with these. Osteopaths may actually be treating two causes of epilepsy – for example, a person may have had birth trauma but not developed epilepsy, only to suffer a bike accident several years later which does precipitate the epilepsy. In this respect, osteopathy is indeed a 'holistic' or 'whole person' treatment.

Osteopathy aims to treat epilepsy indirectly, and to treat the person with epilepsy. By treating the whole body, osteopathic techniques, including soft tissue work and massage, can help take the pressure off the central

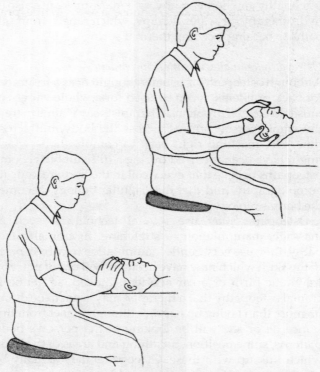

Fig. 4 Cranial osteopathy

nervous system, and osteopaths say this can help reduce the intensity and frequency of seizures.

Chiropractic, often linked with osteopathy, is a separate discipline which works on the belief that disturbances of the spine can impact on the nervous system. A dramatic example of this involves the start of chiropractic, when a Canadian osteopath, David Daniel Palmer, cured his office cleaner of deafness by manipulating his spine. While it may be that a properly aligned spine does lessen strain on the nervous system, and may help normalize nerve transmission of impulses to the brain, some people have reported that this method seems to have triggered seizures. Choose a very gentle practitioner if you want to try this.

Diet

Diet may be the factor which tips the balance when it comes to achieving control of seizures in some people, who find that certain foods or dietary imbalances trigger attacks. Better nutrition, though not a cure for epilepsy, can increase well-being, often in combination with other measures, such as exercise or aromatherapy.

A healthier diet

Make your food your medicine is the often-quoted advice from Hippocrates, and it's true that a better diet does make for better health. But what is a healthy diet exactly?

Plenty of fresh fruit and vegetables is important. By eating more of these, you immediately boost your intake of vital vitamins and minerals, which has added significance if you are taking anti-epileptic medication which may affect your absorption of these. In addition, scientists have now shown that many natural foods are rich in phytochemicals – chemicals which occur naturally in plant foods. Some nutritionists believe that 'superfoods' – foods which have their own therapeutic benefits – can

be as effective for good health as a doctor's prescriptions
(see page 120 for a book on superfoods). For example,
broccoli, like other members of the cabbage or crucifer
family (and green leafy vegetables in general), has been
shown to offer possible protection against some forms
of cancer. It's also thought that the pectin and vitamin C
in apples result in a drop in cholesterol. And garlic is
believed to help combat heart disease, protect against
cancer and – important for those with epilepsy – help
lower stress levels. (Indeed, a healthy diet overall helps
lower stress by making you feel generally fitter and
better.)

As well as fresh foods, try to eat as many whole foods
as possible – as a general rule, the nearer a food is to its
natural state, the better it is likely to be for you. For
example, try porridge oats instead of refined ready-pre-
pared cereals, wholegrain bread instead of white, and
chicken instead of ready-made chicken pie. Eat moderate
amounts of protein, and cut down on fat, sugar and
processed foods.

Some women have more seizures around the time
of menstruation, as described on page 31. Again, extra
attention to diet may help, especially in the week before
your period is due. Try to have small, frequent meals
rather than three larger ones, because your blood sugar
level may drop a few days before your period starts,
which can lead to a vicious cycle of reaching for the
chocolate or other high-sugar foods, sending your blood
sugar level soaring, and then crashing down again. Help
eliminate these blood sugar swings/crashes by making
sure you eat a varied diet, with more whole grains and
whole flours, beans, vegetables, fruits and brewer's
yeast. Try also cutting out (or cutting down on) salt,
sugar, alcohol and caffeine, found in tea, coffee, chocolate
and soft drinks.

Ketogenic diet

Started by a New York doctor in the 1920s, this is a high-fat diet specifically designed for children with epilepsy. It fell out of favour in the 1950s with the introduction of new drugs, but is under new research today for both children and adults.

The ketogenic diet is very high in fats such as butter, cream, eggs and fat meat, while cutting out sugar, bread and other carbohydrates as far as possible. Fats account for 80–90 per cent of the total calories consumed. The body becomes deprived of glucose and develops a condition called ketosis, when it begins breaking down fat cells, producing acids called ketones which are used for fuel and energy. This in turn reduces seizure activity, though it isn't known exactly how it works. One possibility suggested is that the high fat levels help repair the myelin sheaths around the nerves of the brain. Like other treatments for epilepsy, the ketogenic diet must be prescribed and monitored by a doctor.

The ketogenic diet is a demanding, highly inconvenient diet – some people find it too unpalatable to follow, though this can sometimes be overcome by more imaginative use of food. It also has a variable success rate – for several years, some older studies seemed to indicate that it reduces seizures by 40 per cent.

However, the ketogenic diet may have its day yet, as scientists across the USA and Canada are re-investigating it in a cross-cultural study involving several different medical centres. Early results from the Johns Hopkins University in Baltimore, USA, a world-renowned centre for ketogenic diet research and treatment, appear to reconfirm that the diet can reduce seizure frequency and the amount of medication needed. In this study, 22 per cent of youngsters between one year and sixteen years old on the diet for one year remained seizure-free, while 70–90 per cent had seizures cut by half. Researchers are also trying the diet out on adults, where again initial results are promising, reducing seizures by as much as 70 per cent in some.

The diet does have side-effects, such as high cholesterol levels, poor growth, poor weight gain, constipation, kidney stones, vomiting, dehydration, anaemia, loss of minerals in the bones, recurrent infections and lethargy. The diet may also be low in essential vitamins, making careful supplementation necessary. All in all, it really is necessary to talk things through with an informed doctor before you decide to go ahead with the diet.

Case history: Jayne/ketogenic diet

When Jayne wanted to try the ketogenic diet, her neurologist was not very enthusiastic. He thought she was 'doing fine' as she was. Jayne, a twenty-eight-year-old librarian living in the US, disagreed, as she had tried nearly every epilepsy medication going since being diagnosed with epilepsy at the age of ten.

Jayne decided to find out for herself and wrote to the Johns Hopkins University, Baltimore, USA (see page 118 for contact address), who put her in touch with local hospitals. She visited the dietician at one of these, who helped her plan the diet.

'It took a few months to "kick in" but then I gradually found that I was becoming more mentally alert. I found I needed less sleep, and was catching on to other people's jokes quicker. My whole thinking process seemed noticeably speeded up, and my memory was much more reliable.'

After around four months on the diet, Jayne was able to reduce her medication to an all-time low, and now suffers from perhaps one seizure a month.

Nutritional deficiencies

Certain nutritional deficiencies have been particularly associated with epilepsy, and some anti-epileptic drugs deplete nutrients too (so does stress.) Trying to correct deficiencies may be beneficial, though this should be part of an overall nutrition programme. Check out supplements with your doctor first – some anti-epileptic drugs can affect your absorption of certain vitamins and minerals, including vitamins E and B6, manganese, zinc, copper and folic acid. Because your levels of these nutrients may already be lower than average, you may need expert nutritional advice if you want to try vitamin supplements.

Low blood sugar: As we saw on page 30, hypoglycaemic tendencies have been attributed to people with epilepsy, with blood sugar levels falling just before a seizure in an estimated 80–90 per cent of people. If you have seizures if you miss a meal and if you crave sugar you might have a hypoglycaemic tendency. Eat a high-protein diet and have small **non-**sugar snacks every three to four hours.

- **Iron** deficiency (anaemia) is common and people with epilepsy in particular may find themselves prone to it. This is especially true if they suffer digestive troubles as well, in particular diarrhoea.
- **Folic acid** deficiency has also been blamed for seizures, but don't take supplements on your own as some research indicates that this may make epilepsy worse.
- **Vitamin B6 (pyridoxine)** shortage appears to produce epileptic convulsions in some people. Extra doses have helped, though results are very variable. Once you start increasing your intake of vitamin B6, you automatically up your need for other B vitamins, particularly B2 and pantothenic acid, so again this is a matter to discuss with your doctor or a nutritional expert who is also informed about epilepsy. Good sources of vitamin B6 include meat, whole grains and pulses. A vitamin B complex supplement could also help. However, it is important to consult a practitioner when taking this supplement – some people develop neuropathy (abnormality of the nervous system) at incorrect dosages.
- **Magnesium** loss has in extreme cases appeared to

cause uncontrollable epilepsy, in a condition called
nephritis (inflammation of the kidneys), when magnesium is lost via the urine. Magnesium may also
be lost through diarrhoea (see coeliac disease, pages
79–80). Some people have benefited from combining
supplements of both vitamin B6 and magnesium.
Magnesium is found in wholemeal flour, millet, figs,
meat, fish, nuts and pulses (i.e. peas, beans).

- **Calcium** shortage (hypocalcaemia) has been associated with epilepsy in some medical studies (again, see
coeliac disease, pages 79–80), and some research has
found that extra calcium has stopped seizures, even
though the EEG continues to show epileptic activity.
In other words, people with a predisposition to seizures may be tipped over the edge by lack of calcium.
Calcium comes in milk and milk products. Also, take
care to add calcium if you are trying a diet which
excludes dairy products for allergy reasons – other
sources of calcium include nuts, bread, eggs, canned
fish and green leafy vegetables.

- **Vitamin D** is important both in its own right and as
helping the absorption of calcium, and some people
with epilepsy have shown shortages of this vitamin
when tested. It's found in most oily fish and some
animal products, especially in cheese and fortified
milks.

- **Zinc** deficiency has also been associated with epilepsy.
Zinc is important for healthy brain and mental development, and also raises levels of taurine in the brain
(see below). It works best in combination with manganese. Zinc is found in meat and offal, wheatgerm,
nuts, crab, oysters and lentils.

- **Manganese:** While this is still controversial, prelimi-
nary evidence suggests a link between congenital
seizures and deficiency of the trace mineral manganese in the mother's diet. Good sources of manganese
include rice, wholemeal bread, wheatgerm, buck-

wheat, lima beans, nuts, cockles, sardines, blackberries, figs and pineapple.

- **Taurine:** This is an amino acid that helps inhibit neuronal activity, and again some people with epilepsy are deficient in this. **DMG** (Di-methyl glycine) is another amino acid which helps oxygen move round the system and has been shown to bring people out of a fit.
- **Vitamin E** is important for oxygen flow round the body and one trial indicates that it may be an anticonvulsant.

Case history: Anna/taurine

Anna, a twenty-six-year-old music executive, had suffered tonic-clonic seizures for twenty-three years and was willing to try anything. She came across a reference to taurine in an alternative health magazine, and checked it out with her neurologist, who laughed but assured her she couldn't do any harm by taking supplements of taurine.

Anna started with regular taurine from health food stores but didn't feel much difference. 'Then I ran into MegaTaurine and started taking 1,000mg three times a day, along with my regular medication. For six weeks, nothing happened. Then the tonic-clonic seizures just stopped. The absence seizures and myoclonic jerks have reduced but not stopped altogether.'

After four years of taurine supplementation, Anna continues to have reduced seizure activity and no side-effects – though if she runs out of taurine for a few days, she says her convulsive seizures return.

Corrective diet

With so many possible deficiencies to choose from, how do you begin to eat 'properly' – especially if you feel you've always eaten reasonably well before? There is no set epilepsy diet as such which guarantees to correct all deficiencies. Much depends on each individual's requirements. However, nutritional therapists would probably start with a diet based on whole organic food to help stabilize blood sugar and promote good health in general. This would probably exclude common triggers of problems (see list on page 79).

A nutritional therapist would then work out a personal supplementation programme to be used in conjunction with drugs prescribed by your doctor. Improvements would be expected in one to three months.

The allergy factor

Allergies to chemicals, additives and certain common foods have been associated with seizures. At Great Ormond Street Hospital for Sick Children in the UK, a study done on children with migraine and epilepsy found that once allergies had been identified and the culprit foods removed, both migraine and epilepsy disappeared in 78 out of 88 children.

However, don't be too quick to suspect allergy. Allergic-type symptoms can occur if you are lacking nutrients – you may find your health improves if you eat a better diet. An elimination diet can help you decide which, if any, foods are making your condition worse. A classic elimination diet follows some form of fasting to clear the system of allergens, and then foods are gradually reintroduced to see if there is a reaction. This can be a time-consuming process but may be worthwhile if you feel that certain foods are causing seizures.

Interestingly, given the link between seizures and stress, stress can be an important factor in food allergies and intolerance, according to Jill Carter and Alison Edwards, authors of *The Elimination Diet Cookbook* (see page 120). 'When an individual is under stress, the area round the stomach tightens and the flow of intestinal juices is impaired, so that food cannot be properly digested,' say the authors. 'This, in turn, can create more intolerances, thus setting up a vicious circle.'

Suspect substances

What different people react to is highly individual, so probably no list could name every single culprit food. However, certain people have reported that the following foods seem to make them feel more unwell, and even to act as a trigger of seizures:

- White flour
- Red meat
- Dairy produce
- Sugar (sometimes in the coating of medication)
- Foods containing additives
- Tea and coffee
- Alcohol
- Peanuts
- Evening primrose oil – some people have suspected this f triggering seizures.
- Artificial sweeteners – one substance which has come under particular attack is the artificial sweetener aspartame. Research at Arizona State University linked aspartame with epilepsy and reports have been made to the Food and Drug Administration (FDA) of more than 250 seizures after taking it.

Coeliac disease

One particular intolerance which deserves attention is wheat allergy, usually viewed as causing coeliac disease. Several studies (in Jerusalem, Sydney and Italy) have associated coeliac disease with epilepsy. One of the largest of these studies was done by the Italian Working Group on Coeliac Disease and Epilepsy, who found that 77 per cent of their patients with cerebral calcifications and epilepsy also had symptoms of coeliac disease. Coeliac disease may put people at greater risk of seizures because it prevents the absorption of certain nutrients such as iron and calcium (malabsorption syndrome). Nutrients may be washed through the system and then lost in the persistent diarrhoea which is a feature of coeliac disease.

Following a gluten-free diet could help – this means cutting out sources of gluten such as wheat, rye, barley, oats, buckwheat and prepared foods containing these ingredients.

Heavy metal toxicity

Nutritional therapy may also be able to help rid your body of toxicity which has come from a polluted environment. If you live or work in a polluted environment, a nutritional therapist may be able to assess if your body has suffered by using hair analysis to measure the levels of minerals in your body. Any heavy metal toxicity can then be dealt with by chelation therapy, which detoxifies the body using certain vitamins and minerals which wash the heavy metals out of the system. Hair analysis has come in for some criticism as being unreliable, but the general idea of supplementation may be useful if pollution has depleted essential nutrients in your system.

CHAPTER 8

Treating your mind and emotions

While it would be ludicrous to suggest that people are in danger of having a seizure every time they get upset, a person's mental state and emotions can influence whether seizures take place or not. According to Dr Peter Fenwick, consultant at the Institute of Psychiatry, Maudsley Hospital, London, anger and upset are well known to precipitate seizures in more than 15 per cent of people with epilepsy.

The mind and emotions are areas where people can seek help for themselves, and where they do have a certain amount of power to change. This may be through careful and conscious stress management. Other treatments have been designed or adapted to help people with epilepsy, such as aromatherapy and biofeedback, which, though different in approach, both involve a measure of behaviour control techniques. This kind of behavioural therapy has been shown to reduce seizure frequency and intensity in some people, especially if their attacks begin with a recognizable warning. Such techniques may not suit everyone, first because they only apply to people with certain types of epilepsy where attacks begin with a slow warning; and second as some of the mental techniques tend to involve quite a bit of hard work!

Stress

Money pressures, work, relationships – sources of stress abound for everyone, and for some people with epilepsy this has added relevance. A third of all people with epilepsy find they have more seizures in times of stress. A study carried out by the Epilepsy Foundation

---

What is stress and how does it affect the body?

Stress is a natural response by the body to threatening events. When challenged, the body produces a surge of the hormone adrenalin, which increases mental alertness and makes us ready to fight if need be, or to run away – the so-called primitive 'fight or flight' response. This is nature's way of ensuring that the body is primed to respond swiftly to a life-threatening situation, such as a sabre-toothed tiger. In our day and age, however, this response is often inappropriate, and because the stress has no physical let-out, it then tends to build up inside us, often with negative effects on our health.

Hans Selye, a pioneer in stress research, defines stress as 'the non-specific response of the body to any demand made on it, when external demands exceed resources'. He identified three stages of reacting to stress:

- *The alarm reaction* to the source of stress, which activates the nervous system.
- *The resistance stage* occurs as the body acclimatizes itself and adjusts to the stress.
- *The exhaustion stage* which results if stress occurs for too long, and the effects of stress build up – in extreme cases, leading to illness and even death.

Stress – the 'staircase effect'

Stress can build up as the day progresses – the so-called 'staircase effect'. If we do not have time to adapt to the first stress, we hurry on into the next stressful situation still carrying some of this stress. This can be compared to taking another step up on a staircase. If we climb too high, the pressure builds up. Short-term relaxation techniques at different times during the day can prevent the stress from building to an unmanageable level. Different coping strategies and biofeedback (see pages 89–91) help improve these skills.

of Victoria, Australia found that 63 per cent of those who took part believed that there was a relationship between stress and seizure control.

However, this doesn't mean cutting out stress alto-gether – fairly impossible anyway. Some stress is healthy for everyone – it gets the adrenalin going, helps you achieve, and gives a certain zest to life. Also, people vary in their responses to stress. Some appear to thrive on highly stressful lives, while others feel more free in a routine planned to exclude the unexpected as far as possible.

The most important factor is stress as experienced by you, not as perceived by others. Creating a lifestyle which will stand up to stress means a balance between taking responsibility for your life, and accepting your limitations.

Managing stress

The first step in managing stress is to identify as far as possible just what causes stress in your life. Start by writing down your main sources of stress, using the checklists below if necessary.

Just making a list can be very helpful, as it clears the mind and is a visible sign that you are taking a more active role in managing your stress, your epilepsy and your life. Once you've made your list, look through it to see what you can change, and what you have to put up with for now.

Taking an active role against stress

A five-point plan to combat stress:

- **Take control.** Accepting that you are in charge of your life can lessen stress in that you are not dependent on other people, over whom control is limited. By making changes yourself, no matter how small, you can feel more in control.

Checklist: sources of stress
Stress may be triggered by many factors, including:

- Having epilepsy
- Fear of having a seizure
- Fear of other people's reactions to your epilepsy
- Forgetting to take medication/deciding not to take it
- Work, especially if it involves confrontations with boss or colleagues
- Social demands, especially in terms of people you find irritating and/or who make sudden unexpected demands
- Too many interruptions to your routine or demands on your time
- Lack of sleep
- Alcohol
- Unbalanced diet, for example too much sugar, fat, sweets, chocolate, coffee and tea
- Nicotine
- Hyperventilation.

Individual stresses – add your own

Checklist: signs of stress
It's important to realize that stress may be affecting your life well before it actually shows in the form of increased seizure levels. Stress can take various forms, for example:

- Insomnia
- Irritability and explosiveness
- Sleep disturbance
- Digestive upsets such as indigestion or irritable bowel
- Allergies/allergy-related illnesses such as hayfever, asthma and eczema may be worse under stress.

Individual signs – add your own

- **Accept your emotions.** Some people find it hard to acknowledge that they have feelings of anger and fear, sometimes of an overwhelming kind, but coming to terms with your feelings is an important part of stress management.

- **Plan ahead.** Planning ahead reduces uncertainty and indecision, which are also sources of stress. But do allow leeway for unexpected events. Remember, the best-laid plans . . .
- **Use family and friends.** Talk to people who appreciate you for what you are, and who wouldn't have you any other way. A stress-resistant life is lived on your terms, not anyone else's.
- **Respect your own private emotional and spiritual needs.** Take time for yourself, however you do it. Work, social life, even home or love life – there is bound to be a 'you' that these do not impinge on, who sometimes needs to exist independently.

Various stress management methods have been recommended for people with epilepsy, such as art, exercise, music, talking to people and hobbies (research shows that people who are enjoyably employed are less likely to have a seizure). More structured techniques include:

- **Assertiveness training:** This is a technique which helps you honestly communicate your feelings and needs without aggression and underlines the importance of listening to and respecting the other person.
- **Improving self-esteem:** Techniques aim to build up positive thoughts instead of negative ones, and emphasize your own power in creating your self image. They involve actively learning about yourself and taking more control of your life.
- **Anxiety management:** Worrying about the future and possible problems is also stressful. Again, this is a technique which requires you to take decisions on your own behalf, as well as to identify fears and learn how to take control of your life.

Preventing the seizure at the aura stage
Many behavioural methods involve identifying the aura, or warning, which comes before an epileptic attack, and preventing the seizure at this stage. By relaxing, getting breathing under control and concentrating, many people find they can halt a seizure when the aura comes. Meditation may be especially helpful for this (see pages 91–3). Others have developed their own control techniques, which can be as simple as reading a book or lying down. Clare, whose seizures always started with a tingling in her arm, found she could stop them by vigorously rubbing her arm; Jack stopped 'the feeling' by drinking a glass of water; Christopher, a computer designer, would focus on the top right hand part of his computer and think hard about how computers were constructed and all the uses they had. All three found they could halt seizures on many occasions. Finally, research is ongoing into various behaviour control methods which can be used to halt a seizure when the aura starts – in Finland, for example, work has been taking place on a singing remedy, which is obviously distracting, as well as helping control breathing.

Aromatherapy
This is perhaps the best-known and researched complementary therapy for epilepsy, as it has been the subject of much work at the Seizure Clinic at Birmingham University in the UK. In one study, sixteen out of fifty patients became completely seizure-free after a year, and in seventeen people the number of seizures was halved. All had had seizures which had failed to respond to conventional treatment. However, it must be stressed that all the people who took part were committed and enthusiastic, as this technique is only effective with those who are prepared to work at it. Also, it isn't known how long the effect lasts, nor how much practice is needed to keep the response going.

Recognizing that stress, anger and excitement are

prime triggers of seizures, researchers have been using aromatherapy with other methods to produce a state of relaxation in patients which might help them ward off a seizure. Patients are offered a choice of oils and choose the one whose aroma they instinctively like best. Ylang ylang, which has a calming effect, is a particular favourite – interestingly, people being treated for anxiety *without* epilepsy don't usually choose this oil, which has led doctors to speculate whether ylang ylang may have anti-convulsant properties, a question which remains for future research. Camomile and lavender have also been found to be helpful. A few people may need to be stimulated rather than relaxed and so may need a more arousing oil, such as lemon grass.

While still smelling the aroma of the oil, patients are then taught a simple self-hypnosis method, which may be something as simple as raising a hand while concentrating on it to the exclusion of all else. Eventually, people learn to associate the smell of the oil and/or the hypnosis technique with the state of relaxation.

The smell of the oils works on the olfactory (smell) centres in the temporal lobes of the brain, which in turn affect the brain's limbic area, involved in many of the senses, mood control, instinctive behaviour and emotions. The link between the emotions and smell is profound – we all know how a chance odour may suddenly conjure up a situation or person from the past, along with all the feelings from that time. Smell has been used before as a counter-measure against seizures, and it's also important that smell does not become associated with *having* seizures. As you can see, it's a fine balance to achieve, and one which will need sensitive work both from a person with epilepsy and an aromatherapy practitioner.

Using these oils, then, the aim is to create is a 'smell memory' which can be used to ward off an impending seizure. Although people may carry the oils round in small bottles, or use them on a hanky, they don't actually have to sniff the oil every time they feel a seizure coming on – using the right mental techniques, they may be able to 'visualize' the smell, which can be enough to stop a seizure.

Recent research at Birmingham University also suggests that the massage is an important element of the treatment as well. Not only does it teach patients what it feels like to be truly relaxed, but EEG work with oils suggests that the oils may well have a pharmacological (or actual medical) effect which researchers then condition – that is, they teach patients association techniques so that they learn how to associate the smell of the oil with the positive feeling of being able to ward off a seizure.

This treatment may also involve keeping a seizure diary for a few months in order to pinpoint attacks which are related to specific stresses and feelings. Learning to recognize triggers, along with taking more responsibility for treatment, seems vital to the success of this approach.

Although it isn't possible to say how long the effect lasts, there's no doubt that aromatherapy has helped some people control seizures and even reduce medication. This should only be done, however, with the advice of your usual family doctor or epilepsy specialist, not on an aromatherapist's say-so. Like other complementary treatments, aromatherapy is probably best viewed *as* complementary.

If you decide that aromatherapy is for you, consult a properly qualified aromatherapist (see pages 105–14) and make sure you tell the aromatherapist that you have epilepsy – also, if you are pregnant.

Note: Aromatherapy oils are extremely powerful, and certain oils should be avoided by people with epilepsy as they may trigger more seizure activity. These include hyssop, rosemary, sweet fennel and sage, which are thought to stimulate the brain. Rosemary, for example, contains camphor, a known convulsant drug.

Case history: Glynis/aromatherapy

Glynis, aged twenty-eight, started to have attacks when her periods began at thirteen. Initial attacks of hand and arm jerking gradually progressed to convulsions, and primary generalized epilepsy was diagnosed. She was put on sodium valproate, which controlled seizures but made her gain a great deal of weight as she was on a fairly large dose. When she was twenty-six, her convulsions returned even though she was still taking her medication.

Glynis was aware that the return of her seizures was associated with a bad time in her life, in particular a highly stressful relationship. She knew that if she became particularly upset or angry she was very likely to have one of her convulsions. Using a diary for two or three months, Glynis was able to recognize that her tonic-clonic seizures were occurring in association with her anxiety over the problems in her relationship, and was able to recognize when she was becoming anxious. Being massaged with camomile taught her for the first time what it was like to be relaxed and was invaluable in teaching her to discriminate between tension and relaxation. By using the smell of camomile as a counter measure whenever she felt herself becoming tense, she was able to stop her seizures completely; she has been seizure-free for over three years and has regained her driving licence.

Biofeedback

Biofeedback acts on the principle that our thoughts can control our bodies, even processes usually thought to be beyond conscious control, such as our blood pressure, body temperature and the brain's electrical impulses.

Used since the 1960s for stress, biofeedback uses a variety of instruments to measure just how relaxed or otherwise your body is, which 'feed back' the physiological information the body is giving out in terms of lights or bleeps. People with epilepsy may find this kind

of biofeedback useful if they have seizures which tend
to be triggered by stress.

In addition, biofeedback is also used specifically for
epilepsy, when it measures brain activity, which may
then be shown in various forms as a computer game –
for example, as a game showing balls or spacecraft. By
focusing on these images which represent brain activity,
a person can eventually learn to control both the images
and the brain activity.

Around a third of people with epilepsy can sometimes
stop seizures by using mental techniques, according to
Dr Peter Fenwick, consultant at the Institute of Psychiatry, Maudsley Hospital, London, a pioneer in
epilepsy and biofeedback research. At the Institute of
Medical Psychology and Behavioural Neurobiology at
the University of Tübingen, people with drug-resistant
epilepsy found that seizures decreased significantly in
frequency and strength after twenty sessions of biofeedback training. Similar encouraging results were found in
a study at the Department of Psychology in the University of Konstanz, where six out of the twenty-five
patients given biofeedback training became seizure-free.

People do vary widely in their response. This is illus-
trated by a study at the Andrews/Reiter Epilepsy
Research Program, Santa Rosa, California, USA. In this,
83 per cent of patients with uncontrolled complex partial
seizures achieved control by the end of treatment. People
whose epilepsy had started earlier in life, or who had
more frequent seizures, needed many more sessions.
However, even people with the lowest rate of control –
those having daily seizures – achieved 67 per cent, which
suggests that this type of behavioural approach can be
useful in a very wide range of circumstances.

Biofeedback works best with people who experience
partial seizures or secondary generalized seizures that
begin with some kind of warning or aura. Biofeedback
also works better as part of an overall approach to epi-

lepsy management including, for example, seizure diaries and diet.

Hypnosis/Self-hypnosis

Hypnosis can be described as a state of deep relaxation which allows you to access thoughts and feelings which are normally driven away by the bustle of everyday life. This enables you to get in touch with any suppressed feelings of distress, so making it easier to deal with them consciously.

Some people find outside help is needed to do this properly. Hypnotherapy is a specific form of psychological treatment, in which trained practitioners – doctors or non-medical therapists – place you in a controlled hypnotic trance. Many hypnotherapists are also psychotherapists, which means they are better able to deal with unconscious or subconscious feelings once they have come to the surface.

Hypnosis and non-epileptic attacks (NEAs)

Recent research at Stanford University School of Medicine, USA, reveals that hypnosis can be used to identify and even treat people who mistakenly believe they have epilepsy. (See page 21 for more on NEAs.) Neuropsychiatrist Dr John Barry, professor of psychiatry and behavioural sciences at Stanford, estimates that 20–40 per cent of patients examined at Stanford's epilepsy clinic do not have epilepsy. But many patients have both epileptic and non-epileptic attacks.

Hypnosis and self-hypnosis could both be used as a treatment, believes Dr Barry, who has trained several of his own patients in self-hypnosis techniques to trigger seizures, and then stop them.

Meditation and relaxation

The Quakers speak of 'centring down' and this gives a hint of what meditation can achieve – a touching of your

true self, a private escape to your own inner space, a
kind of spiritual airing which leaves you centred and
refreshed. This may mean no more than lying in at week-
ends or sitting on a park bench during your lunch hour.
The important thing is that you are free to drift in and
out of your own thoughts without being impinged on
by outside interruptions, either real or from your own
conscience. In addition, there are several formal meditation methods, one of the best known being
Transcendental Meditation (TM).

Meditation has physiological benefits, too, producing
changes in brainwave patterns, muscular tension, circu-
lation and breathing patterns. A study at the Department
of Physiology, the All India Institute of Medical Sciences,
New Delhi, has shown that people with drug-resistant
epilepsy achieved substantial improvements with the
help of meditation, reducing both the length and frequency of seizures.

Meditation works best if you are physically relaxed,
however you achieve that relaxation – through sleep,
exercise, massage or talking to people. An American
study from the Chicago Department of Health, Illinois,
showed a nearly 30 per cent reduction in seizure frequency after progressive relaxation training, and the
study strongly recommended that this kind of training
be incorporated into clinical practice.

Progressive relaxation training
This well-known technique involves first tensing and
then relaxing muscles from your toes upwards. This
method is designed to help improve your awareness of
your body – many people hardly realize how tensely
they hold themselves for much of the time.

- Lie comfortably on your back in a quiet room. If pos-
  sible, arrange not to be interrupted.
- Clench the toes of one foot hard, then relax them.
- Now tighten and release the muscles of your ankle,

calf and knees, progressing up to the thighs and hips.
Relax after each time you tense a muscle group, and
notice the difference between tension and relaxation.

- Repeat the whole process with your other leg.
- Continue up your body and try to work on muscles
  you're not normally aware of, such as round the eyes
  and on the forehead.
- Try to lie in a relaxed state for at least ten minutes.
  During this time you could also use **creative visualiz-
  ation**, in which you set your imagination to work
  positively on your body and your health. Imagine you
  are in a peaceful, beautiful setting, and then dream
  up some image which sees good health chasing away
  bad – for example, a sky of tranquil clouds gently
  pushing away the dark electric storm which could
  represent seizures. Use this technique to work on other
  problems too, such as headache, or psychological bug-
  bears such as fear.

Case history: Tina

Tina's epilepsy was caused by a cerebral haemorrhage when
the extra blood flow created by her first pregnancy caused
a cyst in her brain to burst. The cyst had lain there unsus-
pected all her life. Tina now suffers from tonic-clonic
seizures, and is trying one of the newer drugs.

Tina finds being ill in itself is something she spends time
worrying about. Hypnotherapy was one of the techniques
Tina found helpful, as she definitely has more seizures in
times of stress, particularly if she doesn't eat or sleep –
which can be difficult with two young children. Lack of
time compounds stress for Tina, who feels she could have
benefited from more time practising relaxation techniques
with trained support, so that she could continue them on
her own.

Counselling and psychotherapy

Problems such as depression and anxiety are common, but can be specifically related to living with epilepsy, such as continuing seizures or self-consciousness at having epilepsy. In addition, there may be problems which are directly due to brain dysfunction, such as stereotyped mood changes before or after a seizure.

- Counselling, though almost mainstream these days, does offer a safe and gentle treatment which can help people cope with stress, whether on an ongoing basis (e.g. long-term sexual difficulties) or in times of crisis (marriage break-up, redundancy). Counselling gives you a chance to talk through your problems with an impartial and experienced listener, who will help you reach solutions for yourself.
- Psychotherapy will help you understand and face up to psychological problems within yourself (avoidance of relationships, ambivalence about commitment, sabotage of career prospects and progress). Psychotherapy is quite distinct from psychiatry, which is a purely medical discipline emphasizing drug treatment of mental problems.

The variety of psychological therapies is immense – co-counselling or re-evaluation counselling, encounter therapy, Gestalt therapy, psychodrama therapy, Rogerian therapy, transpersonal psychology and transactional analysis. If all this sounds rather daunting, there's always laughter therapy, which has been shown to be an excellent way of getting rid of tension and aggressive thoughts!

CHAPTER 9

Energy treatments and other therapies

Many complementary therapies work on the premise that the proper flow of energy or life force is vital to health and that, in illness, it becomes unbalanced or blocked. In traditional Chinese medicine this force is called *qi* or *chi*, in yoga, the Indian word for this is *prana*. Energy therapies aim to re-balance, unblock or stimulate the flow of energy in some way. Energy therapies which have been suggested for epilepsy include:

- Acupuncture (with acupressure and shiatsu) and Traditional Chinese Herbal Medicine (TCHM)
- Flower remedies
- Colour therapy
- Homeopathy
- Reflexology
- Yoga

Acupuncture

Acupuncture often forms part of the work of a traditional Chinese practitioner, and may well be used together with herbal treatment. The needles are inserted at key points along the body to access the twelve channels ('meridians') where *qi* flows through the body. The meridians are said to influence different organs and body systems. Research has shown that acupuncture can stimulate the body to release its own pain-killing hormones, endorphins, so producing feelings of relaxation and well-being.

Can you measure the life energy?

It is not really known whether energy such as *qi* or *prana* actually exists, or whether it is part of a certain way of viewing and describing illness. Some forms of physical energy *can* be measured – for example, the body gives off electromagnetic energy which can be measured in different ways including EEG. A sophisticated computer technique, computerized magnetometry, measures electromagnetic energy up to 50cm from the body's surface. The body also emits thermal or heat energy, as well as sound and light. Experiments have shown that the heart emits forty to fifty times more energy than the brain, and that energy coming from the heart varies according to what sort of mood a person is in. By measuring the exchange on monitors, scientists have also shown that one person transfers energy to another.

However, while it hasn't yet been shown that one person can change another's energy, many complementary therapists believe that energy works at a 'subtle' level – that is, one that isn't possible to measure. So energy treatments may also be called 'treating your subtle body'. Complementary therapists believe that matter is a form of energy, and that our bodies (being matter) are fields of energy which can be altered for the better in the interests of health. What is and isn't possible to measure does change as science advances – for example, quantum physics postulates that matter becomes energy under certain conditions, and vice versa.

Some studies in China have also indicated that acupuncture could be beneficial for epilepsy, and acupuncture is sometimes recommended as a relaxation technique by epilepsy support organizations, who usually stress that there is no proof it works to combat epilepsy. However, one theory is that acupuncture works on the brain, in particular the limbic centre which is connected with moods and behaviour, and is often implicated in epilepsy. A reputable practitioner will not offer acupuncture as a cure, but may offer treatment on a long-term basis with the aim of reducing drugs to the absolute minimum. Certainly, acupuncture has been found to be beneficial for stress and anxiety and so may help those who tend to have more seizures in times of stress.

A traditional Oriental practitioner will take a full detailed history and medical examination (see pages 98–9). The needles, stainless steel and little thicker than a hair, are inserted along the body's channels or meridians at key points to correct imbalances and dysfunctions. Some people feel a tingling or a heavy sensation as they go in, others feel nothing. Many do report feeling more relaxed after a treatment.

Some practitioners are reluctant to use needles because of the dangers associated with a seizure after the needles have been inserted. However, other therapists are happy to use them, for example Dr Wang Fengshan of the Chinese Medical Centre, who says the only instance in which he would not use them is if a patient was showing obvious warning signs of an attack. In any case, there are variations on acupuncture which don't use needles – **acupressure**, which involves massaging acupuncture points; 'cupping' or placing cups on the skin at strategic points; or 'moxibustion' – heat treatment in which a small cone of burning herbs is placed a few centimetres away from the skin. **Shiatsu**, often linked with acupuncture, also involves massage of the key points of the body in order to stimulate the *qi*.

Some people have found that acupuncture has an adverse effect – one man found he had more seizures than usual after treatment and even had a seizure on the therapist's table. In fact, many acupuncturists tell of patients having seizures when needles are inserted – not at all uncommon. Acupuncture should be approached with care by people who have epilepsy; it is certainly not for everyone. This said, it is well known that many natural therapies do make you feel worse before you feel better – the so-called 'healing crisis' or 'aggravation reaction'. This means that symptoms get worse at first and, according to some practitioners, is a sign that the treatment is working. However, if this proves too severe, you should seek further advice.

Case history: James/acupuncture

James was a twenty-two-year-old who had experienced four tonic-clonic seizures, all while asleep at night. This was diagnosed as temporal lobe epilepsy and drug treatment was prescribed. Fearing the side-effects, James decided to try acupuncture and Chinese herbal therapy. 'At least this way I feel I have some control over what is happening to me. I didn't want my life controlled by a drug.'

James also had some dizziness, diagnosed by his neurologist as an inner ear problem. 'This would probably have been been considered a side-effect of the drugs if I had followed that course!' comments James. 'At this point the treatment I have chosen seems much preferable to the mind-numbing and toxic effects of the usual prescriptions.'

Since starting treatment, James has had just one major seizure.

Traditional Chinese Herbal Medicine (TCHM)

This 5,000-year-old therapy, of which acupuncture is a part, is an intricate and complex holistic therapy which requires rigorous medical training from its practitioners, many of whom practise Western medicine too.

TCHM sees health as influenced by our *qi* or vital energy and *xue*, or blood, which must flow freely along the body's meridians or channels. Blockage of these is thought to cause illness; so is any imbalance in the parts of *qi*, called yin and yang. Health is also thought to be influenced by the emotions, body temperature, nutrition, rest and exercise.

A Chinese doctor starts by taking a detailed medical history and gives you a thorough physical inspection which includes looking at your tongue (a traditional diagnostic tool in Chinese medicine), listening to your voice and taking both wrist pulses to check various points believed to give information about the heart, liver and so on.

According to TCHM, epilepsy is diagnosed as phlegm or dampness caused through a blocked heart meridian which disturbs the spirit. Generally, a TCHM doctor will treat epilepsy with Chinese herbs which aim to restore balance within the body, and acupuncture can be used as well. Herbs commonly used for epilepsy include sweet flag root, Chinese senegar root, bamboo shavings or bamboo juice. The aim is to treat the heart, the spleen and sometimes the liver. A strict diet may also be prescribed, for example excluding sugar, fried foods, most dairy products and alcohol.

TCHM practitioners say that, while epilepsy is difficult to cure, TCHM may help reduce, and in some cases stop, the number of attacks. The person may also be able to reduce the dosage of prescribed drugs, though reputable doctors will encourage people to continue taking at least a small dose of anti-epileptic drugs, as epilepsy cannot be controlled with TCHM treatment alone. There is no reliable scientific research to show that TCHM helps reduce the need for drugs, so it is very important that you double-check with your usual doctor before attempting any drug reduction which may be suggested by a TCHM practitioner.

The main dangers are from 'quack' practitioners and poorly prescribed herbs, so always check qualifications. Do not take any herbal remedies unless they have been prescribed for you by a qualified practitioner.

Flower remedies
One of the best-known of the flower remedies are the Bach Flower Remedies, created by Dr Edward Bach in the 1920s and 30s. These use flower extracts, and work on the overall principle of balancing and lifting the

emotions and so improving health – something which may have relevance in epilesy, where a person's emotional state can affect his or her seizure activity.

For example, the Rescue Remedy, a special mix for crises and emergencies, could be used for the after-effects of seizures. This contains clematis, recommended for dreamy states where the mind is disconnected from the everyday world. In general, therapists work on the whole person and look at how he or she reacts to the disorder on both a short-term basis (current emotional state) and a long-term basis (deep personality). So flower remedies might be used as a mood remedy, as well as a treatment for deeper traits. For example, one remedy, scleranthus, is recommended for changes of mood and feelings of being unstable – something which could be a passing state, or embedded in someone's personality.

In recent years, other flower remedies have been developed. For example, Richard Katz, American researcher and psychologist, has created essences from flowers native to California which could have therapeutic effects. And naturopath Ian White has developed the Australian Bush essences from traditional Aboriginal knowledge of how flowers can be used for resolving emotional imbalances. Flower essences continue to be developed by various individuals all over the world, from the UK, America and Australia, to the Amazonian rain forests and the Himalayas. These more modern remedies offer much spiritual and psychological scope. Some are believed to act on the body's energy field or aura, others are said to operate at quantum level, where at a certain point all forms of matter become energy. Still other therapists favour a more traditional 'mind over matter' approach, believing that to treat the person helps resolve the disorder or disease. They may also use a variety of diagnostic techniques, from dowsing – where the direction in which a pendulum swings over a remedy determines whether it's suitable or not – to dream interpretation. While there is no conventional scientific evidence that flower remedies can improve epilepsy, individuals vary enormously in their responses. Sometimes they respond well to combining the flower remedies with other therapies such as counselling, as the flower remedies, by working on states of mind, may raise life issues which need further attention – for example, anxiety or panic attacks could have their roots in job dissatisfaction or an unhappy relationship.

Colour therapy

Some seizures involve the part of the brain which controls sight, and some people experience auras involving visual hallucinations. Colour itself can, in extremely rare cases, play a part in triggering seizures – one person's seizures were triggered specifically by the colour yellow.

In the energy sense, colour therapy is supposed to work on the premise that our bodies emit an aura made up of different colours (the aura that surrounds the body, not the aura that comes before an epileptic seizure). By focusing a particular colour on the body, colour therapy is supposed to change the cell's molecular structure, so improving health.

On a more down-to-earth basis, there is no doubt we are affected by colour. The psychology of colour has received more attention in recent years and it is now known, for example, that blues and greens may be good for stress as they are noted for their calming effect, while certain shades of pink reduce agitation. Some colour therapists say that people with epilepsy should not be subjected to red light, as it is thought to be an irritant colour.

Homeopathy

Homeopathic remedies consist of plants, minerals, metals and other substances; they work on a principle roughly similar to inoculation – that minute doses of substances which provoke a disorder may also cure it. Anecdotal evidence suggests that homeopathy has worked for some people with epilepsy, not for others – results are very fluctuating. Although homeopaths generally stress that time may be needed before any effect shows, some homeopaths report that any improvement in people with epilepsy tends to take place quite soon, and that from then on the improvement continues to build gradually. Again, treatment is strictly individual so it is impossible to generalize about which remedies suit people with epilepsy best. However, some have reported success with calcarea carbonica, which might be prescribed to bring a person's whole energy system into balance (not to treat attacks themselves). Taken from the middle layer of the oyster shell, calcarea carbonica is commonly used for people who deal badly with stress and feel out of control.

Reflexology
Reflexologists believe that our body is reflected in the feet and that massaging the feet at strategic points works on these body parts to improve energy levels and health. For example, the underneath of the big toe next to the second toe corresponds to the brain.

Certainly, reflexology can be deeply relaxing for some people and so again may be of benefit for people whose epileptic attacks seem to be triggered by stress. However, it does need to be used with care in people who have epilepsy, as over-stimulation can trigger seizures, according to the British Reflexology Association. Always consult a reputable practitioner who understands epilepsy and favours a very gentle approach.

Yoga
Yoga, thousands of years old, consists of a series of body postures (asanas) which also influence the mind, and therefore your health. Many of the breathing exercises especially focus on the intake of prana, the life energy mentioned at the opening of this chapter. Many say the exercises leave them feeling relaxed yet exhilarated and

full of go. Yoga can be practised just as a series of physical exercises which form a very effective relaxation technique. Or it can be approached as a mental and spiritual discipline which combines physical postures with techniques such as breathing control and meditation to help achieve inner balance and peace of mind.

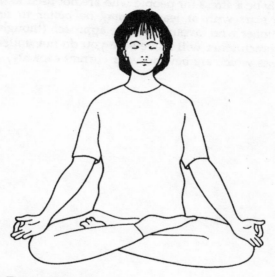

Fig. 5 The lotus position

Regular yoga can reduce stress, and the gentle stretching exercises can help teach the difference between feeling tense and feeling relaxed. The breathing exercises may also be helpful if, as described on page 86, you feel you can sometimes halt a seizure by focusing on your breathing and other mental techniques. Relaxation, deep breathing and postures that massage inner organs can also help with digestive disorders, and so may be helpful for people who have problems with food allergies as described on page 78, particularly if these are associated with stress. Yoga may also improve overall body confidence, which may well be threatened by the sudden loss of control a seizure entails.

There are different kinds of yoga, and some of the more advanced kinds can involve quite complicated and strenuous breathing and stretching exercises which may actually be a stress for people who are not used to them. So, to start with at least, it may be better to find a practitioner who favours a gentle approach (though any good practitioner will make sure you do not undertake exercises which are beyond your current capacity).

CHAPTER 10

How to find and choose a natural therapist

There is no shortage of choice when it comes to natural therapists but it is very difficult to choose from lists of names in telephone directories and advertisements. In many countries, too, not all natural therapists are organized under 'umbrella' organizations, and many certainly don't have neat links with the orthodox medical profession. This means you have to take more responsibility for finding a therapist you feel you can trust. So how do you start the search?

Your doctor

Be prepared for lack of enthusiasm – your doctor may feel obliged to warn you that you will not 'cure' your epilepsy this way. This said, you may be pleasantly surprised at the response you get, and your doctor may be able to suggest a therapist providing your condition is stable. Some health centres have specialist epilepsy nurses who may be able to put you in touch with the very person you need. Your regular epilepsy clinic may also be able to give you some names and phone numbers.

If you need help urgently, you must contact your family doctor or local hospital first. It has already been explained in this book that your condition can decline quickly without the proper treatment, and that, in particular, suddenly stopping prescribed anti-epileptic drugs can be life-threatening.

Word of mouth

Personal recommendation remains the best way of finding a practitioner, from family, friends or work colleagues. They will of course only be able to say what worked for them, and it may not fully apply if they don't have epilepsy (or even if they do, as everyone's epilepsy is different). However, they may be able to suggest someone they feel is trustworthy and caring.

If you have a local epilepsy support group, you may be able to get a recommendation there, too, and it may have the advantage of being to a practitioner who has already worked with people with epilepsy.

Natural health centres

Your nearest natural health centre may be a good source of advice and information. The staff there may even have personal experience of therapies available, and so may be able to offer local recommendations. Certainly they should be informed enough for you to get the feel of the place after an initial chat, and to decide whether it is right for you or not. You can get names from local newspapers, libraries, citizens' advice centres and local information centres. It may also be worth asking around at health food shops, alternative bookshops, beauty treatment centres or health farms if there are any locally. Your pharmacist often has contacts with both conventional and complementary practitioners, so it may be worth asking there too.

Computer network

If you have access to a computer with modem at work or at home, you may be able to get names and addresses of practitioners as well as personal recommendations this way. However, these should still be checked out in the same way that you would check out any recommendation before following it though.

National organizations

National 'umbrella' organizations should be able to provide lists of registered organizations and practitioners. (See pages 116–19 for addresses.) They may charge a small sum for this, and also for postage and packing. Bear in mind that individual practitioners come and go, so even the most up to date lists may not be fully complete.

Checking organizations and therapists

Just because an organization has an impressive name, or a therapist belongs to an organization, professional status is not necessarily guaranteed. So it is a good idea to check out organizations and therapists before undertaking treatment. This isn't just because there are no set standards which apply across the board, as there are in conventional medicine. It's always a good idea to check out anyone you entrust your health to.

Checking therapists may require even more care than usual for people with epilepsy. Complementary therapies specifically for people with epilepsy are new, under-researched and few and far between. So your chances of finding a therapist specializing in epilepsy aren't that good. You are much more likely to find a therapist who has treated a wide variety of conditions including perhaps a few people with epilepsy. So it is vital to make sure the practitioner is informed about epilepsy, to check out any suggested treatment with your regular doctor and to avoid alternative practitioners who suggest you give up your anti-epileptic medication. Liaison between complementary and conventional doctors may be even more important than usual for people with epilepsy.

The first thing to do is check the status of professional associations. A good association should send you clear and simple information about this, though you may well have to ring them up or write to them to get the information you want. Questions to ask include:

- How long has the association been going? (Groups and therapists spring up all the time. Being more established is no guarantee of anything but may offer a track record to help you assess it – on the other hand, new groups may be innovative.)
- How many members does it have? (While size reflects public demand, a smaller group may just mean a new or very specialized one.)
- Is it a charity or educational trust, with a proper constitution, management committee and published accounts? Or is it a private limited company? Charities are regulated and have to work in the public interest – private companies don't.
- Is it part of a larger network of professional organizations? (On the whole, 'lone wolf' groups are more suspect.)
- Does the organization have a code of ethics and disciplinary procedures, and if so what are they?
- How do members gain admission to its register? Are they approved via a school whose head just happens to be the head of the organization too? Be wary: this kind of one-man/woman band means unbiased help may be in short supply.
- Do members have to have proof of professional indemnity insurance? This should cover accidental damage to yourself or your property while you are on the therapist's work premises, negligence and malpractice.

Checking on training and qualifications
If you've got this far but want more information about the qualifications or experience of the people listed, you may find some extra questions helpful:

- How long is the training?
- Is it full-time or part-time?
- Does it include seeing patients under supervision?
- What qualification is awarded?

- What do the initials after the therapist's name mean – membership of an organization, or qualifications gained by study?
- Are the qualifications recognized, and if so, by whom?

Making the choice

Making the final choice is a matter of combining common sense and intuition – that inner feeling that says the person you have chosen is right for you at this moment. Don't forget that the most important part of the whole process is your own resolve to feel better, to have more control over your state of health, and hopefully to see an improvement in your condition. The next most important part is that you feel comfortable with your therapist. As part of an informal chat before you book in, you may want to ask:

- Are you informed about epilepsy?
- Have you treated many people with epilepsy? (A therapist does not have to be expert in epilepsy to be good at what he or she does, but the answer may throw more light on his or her general attitude and competence.)
- How do you regard existing prescribed drug treatment? (A good therapist should not try to tamper with this without consulting your own regular doctor, and one who knows about epilepsy will also know how dangerous sudden drug withdrawal can be.)

What is it like seeing a natural therapist?

There's no one answer to this! Natural therapists come in many different forms – as indeed do conventional practitioners. All have their own styles and ways of being, from the formal to the more relaxed and even unconventional. They range from white-coated individuals with a formal professional manner, to people who are much more unconventional in appearance. They may work from a squeaky-clean clinic complete with receptionist, or a small sitting-room adorned with pictures and plants.

Don't be too reliant on image. While it can indicate status, it isn't the only guide to ability. These days you are as likely to find a quality therapist working from home as from a formal clinic.

Whatever their outward appearance, there are some characteristics common to all natural therapists. These are probably the most important ones:

- An initial consultation will rarely last less than half an hour, and is often longer. By taking the time to ask you all about yourself, your therapist can form a proper understanding of what makes you tick. This means that any treatment will be holistic, that is, of yourself as a person who has epilepsy – not just of the epilepsy by itself.
- You will have to pay for any remedies they prescribe, which they may sell you from their own stock. They will also charge you for their time – though many therapists offer reduced fees for people who genuinely cannot afford the full fee.

Sensible precautions

- Be very sceptical of anyone who 'guarantees' you a cure. No one (not even doctors) can do that.
- Be wary if you are not asked about your existing medication, and be extremely wary if the therapist tells you to stop or change any prescribed drug without talking to your regular doctor first. Never ever give up medication on the say-so of a natural therapist, who may know little about pharmaceutical drugs, and who may not be aware of the particular danger to people with epilepsy in suddenly withdrawing from drugs.
- If you are female, feel free to have someone with you if you have to undress, if the treatment involves touch, or if you just feel more comfortable when

accompanied. No ethical therapist should refuse this, and if they do, have nothing more to do with them.

- Query any attempt to book you in for a course of treatment before you know how you'll respond to the first session. In particular, you should not have to pay fees in advance.
- Don't hesitate to cancel an appointment if you don't like the therapist, the place or the treatment. (Try to give 24 hours' notice if you can, to avoid being charged.)

What to do if things go wrong

Failure to cure you is not an offence. The truth is, it is probably as much of a disappointment to the therapist as to you (though bear in mind that many natural remedies do take a while to work). But failure to treat you with professional care and respect *is* an offence.

A practitioner is in a position of trust – not because he or she has guaranteed a cure, but because he or she has undertaken a duty of care to you. If you really feel this trust has been abused, there are certain actions you can take. Complain to the therapist first so as to give him or her a chance to make amends if possible. Try to establish whether the therapist genuinely was trying to help. If the situation is more serious, then you have no option but to turn your back on the whole episode, or to take further action:

- If the therapist works at a clinic, health farm or sports centre, tell the management.
- If you're not satisfied, tackle the professional body to which the therapist belongs. Don't expect too much, however; many unconventional medicine organizations don't have hard and fast regulations by which members must abide, and so have little or no power over practitioners who break the rules. This is the downside of taking responsibility and going your own 'alternative' way.

- If you still feel you're not getting anywhere, tell everyone about your experience – nothing makes an incompetent practitioner sink faster than a spot of bad publicity.
- In drastic cases when you've been really unlucky and feel you've been the victim of a criminal offence, you can tell the police (but be prepared for the problem of proving one person's word against another's). Likewise, you could also see a lawyer privately for advice; or citizens' advice bureaux may be able to help.

Summary

Despite occasional scare stories about unscrupulous or untrained therapists preying on vulnerable patients, most natural practitioners are serious and reputable people. They have invested time and money in establishing themselves, and may well be practising for strong vocational reasons, or even as a less well-paid alternative to a more secure lifestyle. Despite the myth, there is little real money in it unless the therapist is very busy – in which case he or she is highly likely to be good.

You may need to look round before settling on the right person. It can be disappointing to spend time and energy deciding on a practitioner only to find you don't gel. However, just as you decided to take your health into your own hands, so you can decide to move on – and continue moving on if need be until you find the right therapist for you.

This determination to help yourself get well is perhaps the most important factor in improving your health. Taking control of your own health means taking responsibility for the choices you make. Taking this responsibility, and playing an active part in your treatment, have been shown to help healing.

Remember that no one practitioner can know everything, and that perfection is an ideal rather than a reality. No one but you can decide on a practitioner, and no one but you can determine whether that practitioner is any good or not. Your own feelings will probably tell you this quite quickly.

You may have to shop around to find a therapy and a therapist that suits you, but anyone with epilepsy has a very good chance of finding some form of treatment which helps even beyond what was hoped, improving general health and quality of life. It may have other unexpected benefits, in making you calmer and fitter – and in getting to know someone you trust who can help you monitor your health in the future, and who may even become a friend for life.

In conclusion: Cathy's story

Cathy's story is a clear illustration of how perseverance and the determination to help yourself can be an essential part of improving your health. But her story is also a tribute to how conventional and complementary medicine can work together in accord for better health.

'I was fifteen when I developed encephalitis and, as a result, epilepsy. At first neither my family nor I understood what was going on, as no one ever took the time to explain to us what the prognosis was, and no amount of questioning ever seemed to clarify matters. I was finally sent home and had to take many tablets, though I did still not know why I was having seizures, if I had epilepsy or what side-effects the tablets would cause.

'My teenage years passed in a blur. I went from being an A+ student to one who struggled to pass exams. My memory was damaged, my concentration minimal and my happy-go-lucky character changed to a less confident, reserved one. Things went from bad to worse with more tablets which caused extreme tiredness, erratic periods, hair loss and shakiness – not what you need as an adolescent.

'My consultant did not even know who I was. He became angry if I dared to question him, yet again increased my tablets, and the consultation was over and done with in about five minutes. I was still unaware of any diagnosis and lost more and more faith in this consultant, asked for a second opinion and finally was referred to a centre of excellence for epilepsy. After appropriate investigations (never offered previously) I was given the diagnosis of epilepsy. My seizures were originating from the left frontal region. By this time I was twenty years old – five years of wasted time and inappropriate medication. I was angry, upset and felt very isolated and alone. No appropriate counselling had ever been offered until now.

'With time, I have come to accept and understand my epilepsy more, though I remain angry over the wasted years. I am now married to the boyfriend who saw me through those difficult years and have two children – something I did not think would ever be possible due to my misunderstandings about epilepsy.

'I take only one type of medication, with no side-effects. And finally I have a consultant who takes time to listen, is understanding, answers my questions and basically treats me as an individual. With his help and support, I decided to try aromatherapy as a complementary remedy, and found the mixture of the aroma and the self-hypnosis very useful. Your body starts doing things without you realizing it, making the association between the smell and being relaxed.

'I also pay attention to stress factors such as relationships, work, money and periods – stress does definitely affect me. I found a seizure diary useful in pinpointing triggers – lack of sleep is a terrible one for me. Epilepsy does involve a lot of lifestyle management. You need a very good understanding of your epilepsy, and a proper medical service which allows the freedom to question whether or not a particular treatment is right for you, and which also offers help in deciding which direction your treatment will take next. Even if that includes unconventional treatments such as the use of compementary therapies.' – CATHY F.

Glossary

Absence seizure When a person 'blanks out' for a few seconds.

Anti-epileptic A drug or group of drugs used to treat epilepsy.

Atonic seizure When the person falls limply.

Aura The warning that comes just before a seizure.

Clonic seizure A seizure in which the arms and legs jerk.

Complex partial seizure A seizure affecting part of the brain in which the person's consciousness is affected.

CT scan A modern scan technique using X-ray to give a very detailed picture of the brain.

Electroencephalography (EEG) A method which measures brainwave patterns.

Generalized seizure A seizure involving the whole brain which makes a person lose contact with the outside world.

Myoclonic seizure A seizure involving jerks of the limbs or body.

Photosensitivity When a person reacts to stimuli such as strobe light with a seizure.

Seizure A sudden violent ('paroxysmal') firing of brain cells which affects behaviour and body control.

Simple partial seizure Seizure involving part of the brain in which the person retains consciousness.

Temporal lobe epilepsy A common form of epilepsy involving the part of the brain which controls sensations, memory, taste and smell among other things.

Tonic seizure A seizure in which the person stiffens and falls.

Tonic-clonic seizure A seizure in which the person stiffens, falls and has jerking of the limbs and body.

APPENDIX A

Useful organizations

INTERNATIONAL
International Bureau for Epilepsy
Achterweg 5
2103 SW Heemstede
The Netherlands
Tel +31 23 529 1019
Fax +31 23 547 0119
ibe@xs4all.nl
www.ibe-epilepsy.org/

International League Against Epilepsy
Headquarters Office
Avenue Marcel Thiry 204, B-1200
Brussels, Belgium
Tel + 32 (0) 2 774 9547
Fax + 32 (0) 2 774 9690
www.ilae-epilepsy.org/

UK
British Complementary Medicine Association
PO Box 2074
Seaford BN25 1HQ
Tel 0845 345 5977
Fax 0845 345 5978
www.bcma.co.uk

British Holistic Medical Association (BHMA)
59 Landsdowne Place,
Hove East Sussex,
BN3 1FL
Tel 01273 725951
www.bhma.org

Epilepsy Action (British Epilepsy Association)
Tel +44 113 210 8850
Freephone Helpline: 0808 800 5050
helpline@epilepsy.org.uk
www.epilepsy.org.uk

The National Society for Epilepsy
Chesham Lane
Chalfont St Peter
Bucks SL9 0RJ
Tel 01494 601300
Fax 01494 871927
UK Epilepsy Helpline: 01494 601400

Support dogs (for seizure alert dogs)
The John Fisher Centre
Thorncliffe Park Estate
Chapeltown
Sheffield S35 2PH
Tel 0114 257 7997
Fax 0114 240 2821
sptgods@aol.com
www.support-dogs.org.uk

NORTH AMERICA
Epilepsy Canada
1470 Peel St,
Suite 745
Montreal,
Quebec H3A 1T1
Tel (514) 845 7855/ 1-800 860 5499
Fax (514) 845 7866
epilepsy@epilepsy.ca
www.epilepsy.ca

Epilepsy Foundation
4351 Garden City Drive
Landover, MD 20785
Tel (800) 332-1000
Fax (301) 459-3700
www.efa.org

Montreal Neurological Institute
3801 University Street, Room 285,
Montréal,
Québec H3A 2B4
Tel (514) 398-1980
www.mni.mcgill.ca/library/

Pediatric Epilepsy Center
John Hopkins Medical Institutions
Meyer 2-147
600 North Wolfe Street
Baltimore, MD 21287
www.hopkinsmedicine.org/epilepsy.html

Sheppy's Disability Dogs, Inc
125 Marie Dr.;
Clarksville, TN 37042
Tel (931) 572-0723
Fax (931) 552-4531

AUSTRALASIA
Epilepsy Association (Australia)
PO Box 879
Epping,
NSW 1710
Fax (02) 9869 4122
epilepsy@epilepsy.org.au

Epilepsy New Zealand
PO Box 1074
Hamilton
Tel +64 7 834 3556
Fax +64 7 8343553
national@epilepsy.org.nz
www.epilepsy.org.nz

SOUTH AFRICA
South African National Epilepsy League
PO Box 73
Observatory
7935
Tel 447 3014
Fax 448 5053
info@epilepsy.org.za
www.epilepsy.org.za

Useful further reading

Epilepsy: The Facts, Anthony Hopkins and Richard Appleton (Oxford University Press, 2nd edn, UK, 1996)

The Epilepsy Reference Book, Jolyon Oxley and Jay Smith (Faber and Faber, UK, 1991)

Epilepsy: A Practical Guide to Coping, L Sander and P Thompson (Crowood Press, UK, 1989)

Living with Epilepsy, D Chadwick and S Usiskin (Macdonald Optima, 2nd edn, UK, 1991)

Living with Epilepsy, Peter and Elizabeth Fenwick (Bloomsbury Publishing, UK, 1996)

People with Epilepsy: How They Can be Helped, Mary and John Laidlaw (Churchill Livingstone, UK, 1984)

Understanding Epilepsy, Dr M C Walker and Professor S Shorvon (Family Doctor Publications, in association with the British Medical Association, UK, 1995)

Having Epilepsy: The Experience and Control of Illness, Joseph W Schneider and Peter Conrad (Temple University Press, Philadelphia, USA, 1983)

Epilepsy, Graham Scambler, The Experience of Illness Series (Tavistock/Routledge, UK, 1989)

The Falling Sickness, Owsei Temkin (Johns Hopkins University Press, Baltimore, USA, 1945)

Stigma, Erving Goffman (Prentice-Hall, Englewood Cliffs NJ, 1963)

The Which Guide to Complementary Medicine, Barbara Rowlands (Which? Books, UK, 1997)

The Elimination Diet Cookbook, Jill Carter and Alison Edwards (Element, UK, 1997)

Healing Foods, Miriam Polunin (Dorling Kindersley, UK, 1997)

The British Epilepsy Association provides leaflets and videos on several aspects of epilepsy (see Appendix A for address).
The National Society for Epilepsy also has a video and leaflet information package on epilepsy (see Appendix A for address).

Index